Consent and Confidentiality in the Health Care of Children and Adolescents

Consent and Confidentiality in the Health Care of Children and Adolescents

A Legal Guide

James M. Morrissey
Adele D. Hofmann
Jeffrey C. Thrope

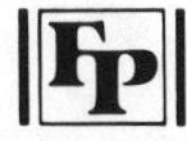

THE FREE PRESS
A Division of Macmillan, Inc.
NEW YORK

Collier Macmillan Publishers
LONDON

The Free Press
A Division of Macmillan, Inc.
866 Third Avenue, New York, N.Y. 10022

Collier Macmillan Canada, Inc.

Printed in the United States of America

printing number

1 2 3 4 5 6 7 8 9 10

Library of Congress Cataloging-in-Publication Data

Morrissey, James M.
Consent and confidentiality in the health care of children and adolescents.

Includes index.
1. Informed consent (Medical law)—United States. 2. Pediatrics—Law & legislation—United States. 3. Confidential communications—Physicians—United States. 4. Children—Legal status, laws, etc.—United States. I. Hofmann, Adele D. II. Thrope, Jeffrey C. III. Title. [DNLM: 1. Adolescent Medicine—United States—legislation. 2. Confidentiality—in adolescence—legislation. 3. Confidentiality—in infancy & childhood—legislation. 4. Informed Consent—United States—legislation. 5. Pediatrics—United States—legislation. WS 33 AA1 M8c]
KF3827.I5M67 1986 344.73′0412 85-28065
ISBN 0-02-921800-4 347.304412

The authors and publisher recommend the use of this volume in accordance with the following statement, which is from a Declaration of Principles jointly adopted by a Committee of the American Bar Association and a Committee of Publishers and Associations:
"This publication is designed to provide accurate and authoritative information in regard to the Subject Matter covered. It is sold with the understanding that the publisher is not engaged in rendering legal, accounting, or other professional service. If legal advice or other expert assistance is required, the services of a competent professional person should be sought."

Contents

Introduction

The provision of health and mental health services is heavily regulated by law, especially where the health care of minors is concerned. The law applicable to these areas has many different sources including the United States Constitution and the constitutions of individual states, federal and state court decisions, federal and state statutes and regulations, and various local laws and ordinances. Some of these laws have nationwide impact; some have impact only so far as the county border. Some laws impose criminal liability for violations, while others provide only a civil remedy, such as an action for damages. As a result there is often confusion and apprehension about "the law": its sources and its effect on health professionals. Health professionals without legal training are understandably wary.

Moreover, the law is not static. In its basic definition, law is an expression of public policy. It is the crystallization of the way society views a given matter or subject at a particular time. Consequently, laws change when underlying public policies change. The evolution of laws governing the relative rights and responsibilities of parents and their minor offspring (as detailed later on) is an excellent example of this process. The movement from nearly complete parental autonomy to the contemporary children's rights perspective largely reflects shifting societal perceptions regarding minority.

Of all legal issues pertaining to the health and mental health care of children and adolescents, the question of whether minors may consent to care is the most troublesome. Most professionals strongly believe that because parents customarily exercise decision making and related negotiations on behalf of minor offspring, the law reposes sole authority in the parents to decide whether a minor may be treated medically, and the minor has no voice of his or her own. Only in the instance of medically incompetent adults is there a parallel situation, but their incompetency is determined on an individual basis.

The general requirement of parental consent for the health care of a minor derives from several important public policies. It is assumed that, as a class, minors lack the cognitive capacity to give informed consent to medical care, and we seek to protect minors by assuring that they are represented by those adults most likely to act in their best interests; that is, their parents. Second, we also assume that it is the natural right of parents, who are responsible for their child's welfare, to exercise dominion and control over a minor offspring and to make decisions in his or her behalf with minimal interference from others. Last, because parents have the duty to support their children, and their financial obligation to a child could be substantially increased if he or she suffered injury as the result of a medical procedure, the parents are given the concomitant right to determine what medical services a child should receive.[1]

When an adolescent reaches the "age of majority," these policy reasons for requiring parental consent fall by the wayside. We presume that, as a class, persons who reach a certain age have the cognitive capacity to make important decisions and are no longer in need of representation by another. It also would be inconsistent with our notions of the autonomy of an adult to permit a parent to exercise control over an adult child. While we may well encourage an adult to consult with family members about important decisions, we nonetheless would not permit the family to exercise a veto power or direct that a particular course be taken against that adult's own particular wishes. Last, because parents generally are not responsible for the financial debts of adult children, there is no economic reason for parental consent for the care of an adult child.

As a class, persons who have reached the age of majority are entitled consent to medical care and the consent of no other person is required.

At the heart of the reluctance of health professionals to treat minors on their own consent is the erroneous belief that it will automatically lead to civil liability. Most often they believe that because a minor is legally incompetent to consent to health care, the physician who treats the minor without parental consent does so without any authority and thus commits a battery, even if the treatment is beneficial.

This belief is greatly exaggerated and is almost never applied by modern courts. We know that the law has always recognized circumstances in which a minor may be treated without parental consent, but these have always been viewed as narrow exceptions to an airtight rule. Members of the health and mental health professions frequently are unsure about when exceptions to parental consent requirements apply. The understandable but unnecessary consequence is the exercise of excessive conservatism, which may well result in greater harm to the minor, when beneficial care is denied or delayed.

A common example of such uncertainty is the management of children with urgent but neither life-threatening nor limb-threatening conditions when parents are unavailable. Parental refusal of treatment constitutes another class of problems; this includes the defective newborn, the rejection of transfusions for religious reasons, or the choice of bogus "miracle cures" over tested therapies in the management of malignancies. The reciprocal dilemma also may be encountered when minors refuse treatment to which their parents have already consented; institutionalization in a mental hospital is a common case in point. Intrafamily conflict of a different sort occurs in instances of child abuse; protecting the child frequently requires the disclosure of information detrimental to the parents. Other relevant concerns surround such diverse matters as the validity of a custodian's consent when the child is in a foster home or institution, and the special consent provisions governing children as organ donors or participants in clinical research.

Minor adolescents, as contrasted with younger children or infants, have their own set of issues, whether claiming emancipation or seeking certain services without parental knowledge even if living at home. Solutions here are somewhat complicated because the law takes both age (e.g., sixteen-year-olds versus six-year-olds) and type of services sought (e.g., treatment for venereal disease versus that for cancer) into consideration. The issue of consent, therefore, must be broken down into subsets depending on the age of the minor and the presenting health need.

Without a doubt, the health professional's concern about who will pay for services rendered to an adolescent without parental consent has also contributed to the reluctance to treat older minors on their own consent, even if the law so permits. Simply demonstrating that a minor may, as a legal matter, consent to treatment is, as a practical matter, only half the solution. Who will pay for the treatment once it is given?

Closely related to the right of minors to consent to health care is the question of whether health professionals are permitted, or even required, to notify parents once treatment is given. We therefore also consider the issue of confidentiality of care given to minors.

Questions of consent and confidentiality not only have legal implications, but inevitably require practical and strategic analysis as well. For example:

- How can the treating professional minimize risk of legal challenge while at the same time ensuring that the minor receives needed care?
- How should the health or mental health record be constructed to provide the best documentation for the optimal protection of all concerned?
- Within the context of health care itself, how can one handle angry parents who have just discovered that their son or daughter was treated without their knowledge, or parents who call to inquire about the purpose of an adolescent's confidential visit?

The questions presented by consent and confidentiality in the health care of children and adolescents are indeed numerous and complex, but, on careful analysis, manageable. It is the purpose of this book to provide as many concrete answers as are available in this sphere, and to provide as much contextual guidance as possible to the clinical practitioner. We depart from the usual legal text, however, in that our interest is not so much how health care providers can protect themselves from being sued, but rather, how best to use the law to benefit patients and enhance treatment options. Our goal is to integrate the legal and medical perspectives in an affirmative manner in service of the therapeutic relationship.

The book is divided into seven sections. In the first chapter we provide background information and underlying concepts that will assist the reader in understanding later discussions of particular situations. This begins with a historical overview which briefly develops an analysis of the assumptions, past and present, underlying most of the laws regulating the health care of minors. We then turn to a "mini-civics" section on the definition of law and its derivations, because much of the delivery of health care to minors is so heavily regulated by law. Last, we define the constitutional right of privacy, which has profoundly affected issues of parental notification, and the doctrine of informed consent, the bedrock of the authority to treat, whether the patient is a minor or an adult.

In chapters 2 and 3 we set forth the law according to patient status (e.g., emancipation) and the law according to patient need (e.g., sexually transmitted diseases). We have attempted to mold these sections to most closely parallel situations that health professionals face on a day-to-day basis.

In chapter 4 we discuss specialized situations. These include: the minor as a donor, the minor as a research subject, parental refusal of treatment, and parental–minor disagreement about treatment.

The fifth chapter examines new directions in health record privacy and analyzes the legal considerations which affect management of patient records. In chapter 6 we address our conclusion that the law not only fails to solve every problem, but also creates some of its own, by recommending a number of practical and pragmatic measures which may help professionals avoid potential legal difficulties.

In the final and in many ways most important section of the book, we set forth an exhaustive state-by-state table of statutes regulating the health care of minors in a manner which keys into the previous sections. Traditionally, articles and texts in this area have not accounted sufficiently for the variations of laws among the states. Simply put, the law of one state may not be the law of another, and nationwide generalizations often are not useful in individual circumstances. A practitioner in a given state, armed with the general interpretive information contained in the text, may turn to the table to determine the specific statutory rules applicable in his or her state. Where we found no specific law, a note is made. Local administrative regulations generally have not been covered but may need to be consulted.

While it is certain that we have not anticipated all the legal questions that may arise in the course of caring for minors, this book offers sound legal orientation for the vast majority of questions. It is designed to serve the needs and interests of health and mental health professionals and those institutional administrators to whom they turn for help. While primarily addressing physicians, because of their high visibility and primary legal accountability, we are keenly aware of the important role of other health care providers. Nurses, nurse practitioners, physician's assistants, psychologists, psychotherapists, social workers, physiotherapists, occupational therapists, and others who are involved in the treatment of children and adolescents will find our discussion attuned to their concerns as well. It is not our intent to meet the needs of practicing attorneys, who generally will have to engage in more extensive legal research in order to obtain detailed information for advising or representing clients. This book, however, can serve as a primary reference and research guide for lawyers and may itself provide sufficient information in many situations.

The authors are especially qualified to provide legal guidance to health and mental health providers. Adele Hofmann is a Board-certified pediatrician specializing in the health care of adolescents. James M. Morrissey and Jeffrey C. Thrope are partners in a New York City law practice and have special expertise in various fields of health law.

In conclusion, we could not have written this book without the dedicated assistance of many individuals. We offer our heartfelt appreciation to all who provided support and contributions. In particular we thank Janet Calvo and Vanessa Merton for their guidance in developing the contours of the book, and Janet Zaleon, Michelle Jacobowitz and Francene Mann for their painstaking research. Last, but not least, we thank Laura Wolff and The Free Press for their confidence and support.

CHAPTER 1

Overview

Historical Perspective: Parent–Child Relationships

The law governing parent–minor relationships is often confusing and inconsistent, and, unfortunately, some degree of contradiction is inescapable. The law is an evolutionary reflection of continuing societal change, but this evolution proceeds in fits and starts—or at least in an uneven manner: some elements are updated and redefined in contemporary terms through legislative, judicial, and constitutional activity while other elements remain archaic and unchanged.

It is also true that the law can no more resolve all conflicts of clashing but equally meritorious rights in a totally fair and equitable manner than can the philosophers and ethicists. When problems are intractable, a judge interpreting the law may choose one of three options: deal with the conflict in an ambiguous manner; select one side as providing for a greater societal or individual good than the other; or sidestep the conflict in its entirety by focusing on factual peculiarities of the case or on a procedural point.

But we may be able to understand these issues if we review significant historical trends. We will seek to demonstrate that the law pertaining to minors in the United States has changed dramatically from early colonial to contemporary times, yet elements from each evolutionary phase persist and are very much operative today. In many respects these are more than archaic residues and reflect significant, irreconcilable differences of opinion among legislators and judges as to the basic presumptions governing the relative rights and responsibilities of parent and minor child. In this section, we highlight significant trends, helping the reader to understand the variable, and sometimes inconsistent, assumptions which underlie the law in this area.

Codified law in early colonial America encompassed a "parental sovereign" approach insofar as children were concerned. Derived from seventeenth and eighteenth-century English law, statutes defining intrafamily relationships tended to recapitulate prevailing European social structures, which were aristocratic and hierarchical in form. Children had no constitutional or protective rights of their own, and parents had almost absolute autonomy in respect to their minor offspring and hence almost complete control.[1] Exceptions were limited to criminal acts against the child, and in certain limited instances, to legal mandates insuring that children attended church. Parents were entitled to the child's absolute obedience as well as to the "fruits of his labor." A law in seventeenth-century Massachusetts provided that any child over the age of sixteen who struck his parents or overseers could be put to death unless it could be proved that "the parents have been very unchristianly negligent."[2] While there is no evidence that any youth was indeed subjected to this penalty for cause, the existence of such a law is a reflection of the colonial attitude toward children.

This perspective, moreover, was not simply the remains of European tradition. A highly controlling attitude toward children also responded to the interests of colonial times. Our current view of the nurturant needs and familial role of children is very different from that of Americans two hundred years ago. The modern household cannot be compared to that of the eighteenth century, so often cramped, crowded, and eclectic in composition: comprised of apprentices, indentured servants, and assorted other persons as well as natural children. While wives were constantly giving birth, high infant mortality rates severely compromised infant survival.

Reciprocally, the substantial risk of maternal death attendant on childbearing and the frequency with which fathers succumbed to accidents and wars resulted in many children being orphaned early in life, to be taken in by relatives or neighbors. Even when parents survived, it was commonplace for youngsters to be sent from their own home, if it was crowded and lacking sufficient food for all, to board out and work in another household less amply "blessed."[3] The role of children was largely economic, determined by the work they could perform at home, on the farm or in cottage-based industries, or by the money they could earn elsewhere, making a significant and necessary contribution to their often marginally solvent family. Education beyond learning a trade, and being sufficiently literate to conduct day-to-day business and read the Bible, had little utility and scant societal support. An early work role for children was far more to the point.

There also was a philosophic view that children had a duty to repay parents for food, clothing, and nurture through respectful obedience. Indeed, many age-old laws permitting parents to claim the wages of their children survive today.[4] While parents also bore a duty to raise their children properly, this duty was not seen in today's developmental perspective. The emphasis was on the future and on molding the child to grow up—for the good of the community—into a God-fearing, self-supporting citizen. The parental sovereign perspective, then, was responsive to a time when everyone, child and adult alike, had to work to survive; and when the moral dimension was often governed by a rather stern puritanism aimed at exorcising frivolity, waywardness, and intemperate behavior to the end of personal salvation. Thus, the role of children was quite consistent with colonial life and not at all as exploitative or as punitive as we might tend to interpret it in contemporary light.

During the nineteenth century and into the early twentieth century, however, a number of events created a wholly new conceptualization of childhood, with parental sovereignty giving way to a view which placed far greater emphasis on the child as a dependent, immature being with specific age-related needs. One major influence was the introduction of psychological concepts leading to a developmental orientation; emotional nurturance during the tender years became as important as attention to economic and spiritual preparedness for the future if the child was to grow up well.[5] Second, industrialization, urbanization, and immigration led to the extensive use of children in labor under highly adverse and exploitative circumstances, pricking an emerging social conscience.[6] In addition, advancing technology required increasingly skilled workers, and in consequence, demanded a public policy supporting extended and compulsory education.

The effect was the evolution of the "child welfare" perspective. While parents continued to enjoy wide latitude in rearing their offspring, restraints were now imposed. The state gradually introduced certain boundaries in protecting the child which parents could not transgress. Most notable were compulsory school attendance laws and severe restrictions on both kind and duration of labor. Parents could no longer look to their offspring solely as a source of family support. Nor could parents maltreat their children; the state would now step in and remove maltreated children from parental custody. For the first time, the state recognized the child's needs as separate from family needs and interests. Indeed, the state replaced parents as the final arbiter of child welfare parameters.

It should be noted, however, that the courts were and continue to be quite reluctant to contravene parental rights unless the circumstances warranting such a step are patently clear.[7] The law—and society—remain committed to the centrality and importance of the family unit, maintaining the view that in general, the best interests of the child are best served through parental representation and that this relationship should be disturbed only by exception rather than rule and only for significant cause.

While the child welfare laws enacted in the late nineteenth and early twentieth centuries gave children definitive protections which they had not previously had, it is important to note that minors had not gained the right to self-determination. Protective rights are not the same as affirmative civil or constitutional rights, and minors continued to be denied these. All that had happened was that the state had elected to place itself in the parents' stead (*parens patriae*) when the latter were found wanting. The basic premise that children lacked constitutional rights and protections prevailed. One or another adult continued to decide what was in the child's best interests and the child continued to have no say of his own.

It took the passage of a significant number of years for yet another shift to occur, a shift which is very much at the forefront today. Although the Constitution previously had been interpreted to protect children, in 1967 the Supreme Court clearly endowed minors with the right to claim, for themselves, at least some constitutional protections. This landmark case, entitled *In re Gault*,[8] revolved around Gerald Gault, a sixteen-year-old Arizona schoolboy, who, with a friend, had made an obscene phone call to a neighbor. The neighbor reported him to the juvenile authorities, who then found Gerald in need of rehabilitation and remanded him to the state training school for a period of time which could have been more than five years—or until the boy's twenty-first birthday. Gerald was not given notice of the charges against him, was not allowed to cross-examine his accuser, and was not provided with representation by an attorney. The Supreme Court found that the juvenile court procedure was unconstitutional, and ruled that minors charged with delinquency must be afforded most of the constitutional safeguards afforded adults.

Recently, however, the Supreme Court permitted the use of preventative detention of minors accused of delinquency on the basis that it protected the juvenile from committing crimes prior to trial, and, because the parent has custody over the minor anyway, the detention was merely a transfer of that custody.[9] Note the subservience of the minor's constitutional rights to the parental sovereignty perspective (power of custody) and the child welfare perspective (protecting juveniles from their own improvident acts).

In 1969 the Supreme Court also supported the right of minors to free speech.[10] It refused to uphold the action of an Iowa school principal in his suspension of three young teenagers who persisted in wearing black armbands (in protest against the Vietnam war) on the school premises against his orders. The Court ruled that students were as entitled to the expression of their views as were adults and that the public statement of student opinion could not be constrained unless it would prompt significant classroom disruption or otherwise interfere with the educational process.

This new "minors' rights" perspective continued to expand over the ensuing years, largely in the realm of due process in schools, juvenile justice, and sex-related health care. This change was not without exception; a number of rulings continued to fall into the "child welfare" category, with decisions based on what was best for the minor as decided by adults.[11] It was clear, however, that the law no longer rigidly held to the old position that individuals had no constitutional rights of their own until majority. A new perspective had been introduced under which children enjoy at least some constitutional rights without regard to their age.

These directions were soon to culminate in a particularly dramatic turn in the evolution of "minors' rights." To grasp fully how this came about, it is important to recall the 1973 Supreme Court ruling establishing the right of a woman and her physician to be the sole determiners of whether she should have a first-trimester abortion—a ruling which was recently extended into the second trimester.[12] This was a capstone decision following a series of decisions which collectively established a woman's right to privacy (that is, freedom from state intervention) in matters pertaining to fertility. We thus come to a crossroads in which minors were increasingly exercising constitutional rights of their own and in which a new right of privacy for women relative to their control of fertility had been established.

In 1974 the right to privacy in deciding on an abortion was extended to minors, and laws requiring prior parental consent were ruled invalid as unconstitutionally—and impermissibly—investing a potential veto power in a third party (or someone external to the patient–physician dyad).[13] Later decisions have established that parental or judicial consent may not be required before most minors may obtain abortions.[14] (See "Abortion" in Chapter 3.)

Today laws governing minors often reflect all of the three trends described above. The above overview is offered to provide a basic understanding, in analyzing a particular statute or judicial decision, of which of the three presumptions—parental sovereignty, child welfare, or minors' rights—is operative. It is also possible for two or even all three to be operative at the same time. Much of the inconsistency and confusion surrounding current law pertaining to minors' health care can be attributed to this fact, since each perspective contains presumptions which are potentially at odds with those of the other presumptions.

Most health care encounters with minors proceed without dilemma, as parents usually exercise familial sovereignty in an altruistic manner with every concern for their child's welfare and individual rights. Conflict and confusion do arise often enough, however, to haunt the health care professional. We seek to guide the professional in choosing the course which best serves the minor patient's needs in such instances. Where a particular area presents constitutional concerns—for example, sterilization, contraceptive care, or commitment of a minor to a mental hospital—we have set forth a specific discussion of the relevant issues in the most appropriate section of the text.

Definition of Law

Before discussing in detail the legal regulation of consent and confidentiality in the health care of children and adolescents, it will be helpful to review the construct of "the law" in general: its sources and workings.

Constitutional Law

The United States Constitution is the ultimate expression of public policy, and, as such, is the "supreme law of the land." It sets forth the structure of the United States government. It also contains principles which establish the limits of government action, as are particularly addressed in those amendments, commonly referred to as "The Bill of Rights," in which the Constitution guarantees freedom of speech, freedom of religion and assembly, due process, etc. The action of any legislative body may not conflict with a provision of the Constitution. If a court determines that a particular statute is in conflict, the court must declare that statute unconstitutional and unenforceable.

For example, the statutes which absolutely prohibited a woman from obtaining an abortion were declared unconstitutional because they violated a woman's constitutional right to privacy to exercise control over her own body.[1] Courts, however, generally presume laws to be constitutional and will not declare a law to be unconstitutional if their decision could rest on a narrower, nonconstitutional ground. Also, each state has a constitution with which state laws must conform.

The Constitution is interpreted by the courts when actual cases and controversies arise. Courts may not render advisory opinions or interpret constitutional principles on purely hypothetical questions. Moreover, these interpretations are not immutable and may be redefined with the passage of time, often reflecting shifts in public opinion. In the nineteenth century, for example, "separate but equal facilities" for black and white citizens were deemed constitutional.[2] But in the 1950s this same position was declared unconstitutional, reflecting major shifts in societal attitudes about discrimination.[3]

Statutes and Regulations

The second source of law is statutes and ordinances enacted by various legislative bodies including the United States Congress, state legislatures, and local governmental bodies. The authority of a statute or ordinance extends only as far as the authority of the enacting body. Statutes passed by Congress have nationwide effect, but those passed by the legislature of a particular state have no effect outside that state's boundaries. Most statutes dealing with the delivery of health care to children and adolescents are state laws. As such, they have no effect beyond the particular state in which they were passed. With the exception of certain Constitutional protections in sex-related health care, each state is generally free to enact laws as it sees fit regarding minors' ability to consent. In order to give maximum guidance to the practitioner, we have included a table, setting forth for each state the relevant regulating laws. (See the Appendix.)

Frequently, a legislature enacts a statute which is only a skeletal outline of an intended solution to social problems. For example, the Congress might enact a statute which states as a policy that the federal government should assist in eradicating drug abuse. The task of filling in the details is often left to the executive branch and its appropriate administrative agency. The United States Department of Health and Human Services is customarily given authority for promulgating and implementing regulations for congressional health care appropriations enactments. A similar relationship exists between state legislatures and departments of health and social services. Administrative regulations have the force of law but may not go beyond the authority granted by the legislature nor conflict with the statute's wording or purpose. If they do, a court may declare them invalid.

A recent example of this involved the Title X program, which provides funding for family planning services, including those for minors. Congress, after a substantial and often bitter debate, passed a statute which stated that family involvement should be *encouraged* in the delivery of these services to the young.[4] The Department of Health and Human Services took a much more restrictive position and issued regulations which *required* such involvement. These regulations were declared invalid by the courts because they conflicted with the clear congressional intent behind the statute upon which the regulations were based.[5] Similarly, state and local regulations may not impose requirements which go beyond the limits imposed by the U.S. or state constitution or enabling statute. For the most part, state and local regulations have not been included in the statutory summaries of this book, but they are influential, and practitioners should consult them when appropriate.

Cases Before the Courts

Court decisions constitute the third source of law. There may be no definitive statute governing a given situation, or, if there is an applicable statute, it may be vague, archaic, or ambiguous and require interpretation. In addition, there may be many different statutes within a given jurisdiction, each of which has a bearing on a particular case. Here, too, guidance by the courts is needed. It should be noted, however, that court interpretations may not be the final word. If the legislative body which enacted the statute in the first place disagrees with a court's interpretation, it can subsequently amend the statute or pass another which more accurately reflects its intent. A state legislature, however, may not override the requirements of the U.S. Constitution or federal statutes or regulations.

Like legislative systems, court systems parallel our overall governmental structure. The federal court system consists of the United States Supreme Court together with district and circuit courts located in various parts of the country. District courts are first-level, or trial-level, courts, while circuit courts hear appeals from lower court decisions. The Supreme Court, as ultimate guardian of the Constitution, hears and decides selected cases appealed from federal circuit courts or the highest state courts.

State court systems vary in their precise structure and in the titles applied to different levels. But all are organized in a hierarchical, pyramidal manner. At the base are the lower, trial-level courts. Then come one or two intermediate levels of appellate courts. The system culminates in a single highest state appellate court, sometimes referred to as the state's supreme court or court of appeals.

There also are entities called administrative law courts which are forums set up by statute to deal with particular issues involving an administrative agency's regulations. These bodies frequently are asked to determine how such regulations should be applied when they are ambiguous or unclear relative to a given situation. Decisions of administrative law courts usually may be appealed.

Each court may hear only certain types of cases. Commonly, these restrictions are statutorily derived. Some courts, for example, hear only criminal cases, some only civil cases, while others are limited to petty claims. The extent of the impact of a court ruling also is restricted. The ruling generally is binding on the parties immediately involved in the case, or the plaintiffs and defendants, unless appealed to a higher court and overturned. A ruling's broader application depends on the nature of the case and its implications for establishing "precedent." Precedent means that if a rule of law has been established in one case, it must be followed in all subsequent cases provided two conditions are met. First, the circumstances of the initial case must be sufficiently analogous to those of the later case in which precedent is to be applied as to involve the same questions. This is not always easily established, and the similarity or dissimilarity of cases is frequently a matter of substantial debate. Second, the court rendering the initial decision must have some authority over courts hearing later cases. The highest court in one state need not follow the precedent of the highest court in another state; but within the same state, a lower court must abide by the past rulings of a higher one.

Cases coming before the courts are of two general categories: criminal and civil. In a criminal case, a governmental entity always is a party to the process and seeks to prosecute an individual or group of individuals, as defendants, for alleged violation of criminal laws. If found guilty, the defendant may be imprisoned, fined, or both. Criminal cases usually are prosecuted by district attorneys, state attorneys, or United States attorneys in the name of "the people." A case entitled "The People v. John Doe" would indicate that it involved a criminal matter.

Civil cases cover a wide range of other situations. Commonly these are cases in which two private parties are seeking the intervention of the court to resolve a difference between them. A governmental entity, however, may also be a party here. The party initiating the case is known as the plaintiff or petitioner; the party against which claims are being made is called the defendant or respondent. Civil cases seek to declare the relative legal rights of the opposing parties; or, through force of law, to stop one party from engaging in certain kinds of activities; or to award one party money to compensate for some wrong he or she has suffered at the hands of the opposing party. Punishment through imprisonment or fine is not an objective. A malpractice action is a civil case.

It is important to keep these concepts in mind when considering the law relative to minors' health care. The vast preponderance of claims made against health providers, either for negligence or for failing to obtain parental consent, are not criminal but civil in nature, limited to considerations of liability for damages and monetary awards for wrongs done.

Law and the Principles of Medical Ethics

While it would greatly simplify our professional lives if law and ethics* were identical, this is not the case. As we have already noted, laws derive from state and federal constitutions, statutes (and their attendant administrative regulations), and court decisions. Principles of ethics for the various professions derive from nongovernmental sources, particularly voluntary organizations of professional peers. Their intent is to define appropriate standards of conduct for members of the profession. The ethical principles are generally meant to protect patients by assuring a common level of professionalism among practitioners. The differences between the ethical principles of a profession and law are well expressed in the preamble to the *Principles of Medical Ethics* of the American Medical Association, also used by the American Psychiatric Association.

> The medical profession has long subscribed to a body of ethical statements developed primarily for the benefit of the patient. As a member of this profession, a physician must recognize responsibility not only to patients, but also to society, to other health professions, and to self. The following Principles, adopted by the American Medical Association, are not laws, but standards of conduct which define the essentials of honorable behavior for the physician.[6]

Perhaps the most salient difference between ethics and law is the consequences which obtain should either be violated. If one violates a law, liability may result, either civil or criminal. The violation of an ethical principle, however, is not subject to criminal or civil sanctions, although other punitive actions may result. The offending member may be suspended or expelled from his or her professional society. Disciplinary action may be taken by a local pro-

*By "ethics" we refer to the principles of ethics enacted by the various professions, and not to ethics as an academic discipline.

fessional licensing agency, even leading to suspension of licensure if the lapse in conduct is particularly egregious.

Medical ethics may even conflict with existing laws which are inconsistent with the patient's best interests. Under these circumstances, professionals may feel themselves bound to seek legal change. For example, many of the lawsuits mentioned earlier that established a woman's right to privacy and freedom from state intervention in matters of sex-related health care were litigated by physicians, some of whom risked criminal prosecution rather than obey a law they believed contrary to their patients' best interests and unjust or unconstitutional.[7] Thus it is quite conceivable that a professional could violate a law without being guilty of unethical behavior.

The converse also may be true. A professional could well treat a patient adequately and without inflicting specific harm, and thus be free from legal sanction; yet this treatment could be unethical. Obesity clinics employing questionable treatment with stimulant drugs are one example. Another is the performance of surgical procedures on an outpatient basis when safety and the patient's best interests commonly dictate this be done in a hospital setting; some professionals would include home birthing in this category.

Finally, although professional ethics do not constitute law in and of themselves, they often suggest the law's future evolution. Courts, in determining a clinician's liability, will certainly be profoundly influenced by what his or her peers, as a class, deem appropriate ethical behavior.

In this book, we have limited ourselves to discussing the law. Questions regarding ethical behavior or dilemmas are beyond our scope. But this is not to say that ethical issues should be ignored or that legislative or judicial correction should not be sought when law and ethics conflict to the detriment of the patient.

Informed Consent

The concept of informed consent is a vexing one for physicians, patients, and courts alike. Its origin is recent, and today its legal definition remains in flux and varies from state to state. We do not intend to discuss this highly complex issue at length, but we will highlight selected aspects as they apply to minors. For greater detail, we refer the interested reader to two excellent books: *Informed Consent: A Guide for Health Care Providers*, by Arnold J. Rosoff, and *The Silent World of Doctor and Patient*, by Jay Katz.[1]

The doctrine of informed consent finds its roots in the most fundamental and basic rights of free people: the inviolability of the human body and the right of a person to exercise complete dominion over his or her own person. These rights were well expressed in 1914 by Judge Benjamin Cardozo before he became a Supreme Court Justice. He wrote, in *Schloendorff* v. *New York Hospital*: "Every human being of adult years and sound mind has a right to determine what shall be done with his own body; and a surgeon who performs an operation without his patient's consent, commits an assault, for which he is liable in damages."[2]

The facts before Judge Cardozo were quite shocking and are illustrative of a time when physicians felt they had free rein to treat a patient as they deemed beneficial, regardless of the patient's wishes. In *Schloendorff*, the patient was admitted to the hospital suffering from a stomach disorder. The treating physician discovered a lower abdominal mass and advised the patient that its nature could only be properly determined under ether examination. The patient consented to the examination but expressly ordered the physician that an operation was not to take place. While the patient was unconscious, a fibroid tumor was discovered; the physician removed the tumor in contravention of the patient's command. The case, however, did not address the proposition that a consent must be "informed" as that term is used today, but, rather, the proposition that patients alone have the right to consent to medical treatment—a right that cannot be arrogated by the physician.

It was not until 1957 that the courts began to recognize that patients have not only the right to consent to medical treatment but the right to be given information about treatment allowing them to meaningfully exercise their choice; at the time this was a startling development, one which was denounced by many physicians as an incursion upon their medical judgment.[3]

Over the past thirty years, there has been much judicial and legislative activity regarding the extent and nature of information which must be imparted to the patient for the consent to be informed. In Rosoff's *Informed Consent*, after analyzing the case decisions and statutes in this area, the following are identified as required items about which the patient must be informed:

- The patient's diagnosis (i.e., the patient's condition or problem).
- The nature and purpose of the proposed treatment.
- The risks and consequences of the proposed treatment.
- The probability that the proposed treatment will be successful.
- Feasible treatment alternatives.
- The patient's prognosis if the treatment is not given.[4]

The manner in which the informed consent is obtained must be adapted to the ability of the patient to understand. Thus the requirements for informed consent are probably more troublesome for the patient who has limited cognitive abilities. The physician must take more pains to ensure that the consent is indeed informed. If the patient is of such limited ability that he or she cannot possibly understand the treatment (and no emergency exists), the physician should not proceed with treatment until consent is obtained from a family member or other authorized guardian. (But see chapter 3 for discussions of abortion, sterilization, and organ donation; when these procedures are involved, the right of a family member to substitute consent for an incompetent individual is limited.)

The requirement that a physician obtain the informed consent of a patient before treatment has been subject to several limitations which enable the requirement to be waived altogether. The most common limitations are:

- A risk which is common knowledge (i.e., an injection) need not be disclosed.
- The patient affirmatively represents that he or she does not want the risks disclosed and will proceed with the treatment without such knowledge.
- An informed consent was not reasonably possible (i.e., an unconscious patient required emergency care).

- Disclosure of the risks would substantially and adversely affect the patient's health (therapeutic privilege).[5]

The issue of informed consent and minors can be confusing because of the overlap of the right of minors as a class to give legal consent (to treatment for a sexually transmitted disease, for example) and the developmental ability of an individual minor to give informed consent (presuming the legal competency to do so). If a minor is not legally entitled to consent to health care (e.g., a seven-year-old who requires nonemergency surgery), the issue of informed consent does not arise. In this situation, the physician looks to parents for informed consent on behalf of their minor child, and in some respects, such a consent may need to be more complete. At least one court has held that disclosure to the parent of a minor might be more extensive because the exception of therapeutic privilege, defined above, is not available when disclosure is made to a person other than the patient.[6]

But, as we will show throughout this book, minors may consent to many forms of health care on their own, and issues of informed consent are therefore important. It is interesting to note, however, that we were not able to find a single reported decision which held a physician liable for treating a minor for his or her own benefit without obtaining informed consent. Given the difficulties of proving that a patient's consent was not informed and the the person suffered harm as a result, very few individuals, even adults, have successfully sued physicians on the basis of this theory.

The doctrine of the "mature minor" must serve as our guide in understanding the issue of a minor's consent. The "mature minor," almost by definition, sets out the contours of informed consent from young people. This doctrine is discussed in detail in chapter 2. Briefly, it permits a minor to consent to medical care independently, even if still living at home, as long as he or she is sufficiently mature or intelligent to understand and appreciate the benefits and risks of the proposed treatment.

The information that must be disclosed to a minor in obtaining informed consent is the same as that required for adults. The difficulty lies in assessing whether a minor indeed can understand and appropriately weigh this information, and thereby consent in an informed manner. The issue, however, should not be overcomplicated: what does the physician look to in determining that he or she has obtained informed consent from any patient? One looks to the patient's age, the manner in which he or she conducts himself or herself in the health care setting, the degree of intelligence evidenced in the questions he or she asks, and other such factors indicating a reasonable competence in decision making and self-reliance. Albeit subjective, these factors should guide the professional in determining whether an individual, adult or minor, can or cannot reach a reasoned decision to undergo the proposed treatment.

In cases where the courts have applied the mature minor doctrine, they have regularly found such minors capable of giving informed consent. For example, in *Lacey* v. *Laird*[7] an eighteen-year-old minor (when the age of consent was twenty-one) was found fully able to understand and consent to a simple operation involving plastic surgery; in *Younts* v. *St. Francis Hospital and School of Nursing*[8] a minor was permitted to consent to minor surgery because she was of sufficient age and maturity to know and understand the nature and consequences of the procedure; and in *Bakker* v. *Welsh* a minor was found competent to consent to have a tumor removed because he was "almost grown into manhood."[9]

Thus, in determining whether the minor is of sufficient ability to give informed consent, the physician should look to the following:

1. The age of the patient.
2. The person's intellectual (cognitive) maturity.
3. The ability of the minor to understand the items of information required by the doctrine of informed consent.[10]

If minors, as a class, are legally permitted to consent to a particular form of health care, but an individual minor is not of sufficient maturity to give informed consent, treatment cannot take place. However, it rests with the provider to assist a minor by setting forth the requisite information in terms the minor is familiar with and are appropriate to his or her level of learning, vocabulary and comprehension skills. Technical and highly abstract explanations suitable for adults may not be so for adolescents. When information is conveyed in age-appropriate terms, however, the adolescent may well be able to make a reasoned decision, although at first glance it may have appeared otherwise.

Overall, it is clear that where the courts have viewed minors as mature enough to consent to medical treatment, the procedures involved have been relatively uncomplicated and have been recommended for the minor's own benefit (thus excluding tissue or blood donation). Where the procedure is complex, or high-risk, or for the benefit of someone else, the consent of a legally responsible adult should be obtained if possible.

Right to Privacy and Parental Notification

Presuming the minor has given consent to health care, does the health service provider have to notify the parents of treatment? In any discussion of the delivery of health care to minors, the question of minors' rights to keep treatment confidential from their parents naturally follows that of their ability to consent to that treatment. Even though an individual may legally consent, it does not necessarily follow that the patient, whether minor or adult, is the sole determiner of where or to whom information about the treatment may be disclosed. Such issues are governed in large part by the relative weight of societal interests versus individual privacy rights pertaining to the receipt of a particular form of health care at hand.

The constitutional right to privacy is simply the right of individuals to be "left alone"; the right to make certain personal decisions free from the interference of others, including the state. While not set forth specifically in the United States Constitution, the right to privacy is nevertheless deemed to be one of the most sacred rights of free peoples, deserving of the utmost protection. The right to privacy, however, does not extend to all areas of activity, but only to those areas which are so fundamental to our concepts of liberty and justice that they receive constitutional protection. The right of privacy does encompass such important issues as a woman's decision to terminate or continue a pregnancy,[1] or a couple's decision on whether or not to have children or practice contraception,[2] or one individual's decision to marry another individual (presumably of the opposite sex).[3] However, it does not protect persons affected by laws requiring physicians to report the names of those for whom certain controlled substances, such as narcotics, have been prescribed.[4] Here the state's interests are deemed more important than an individual patient's confidentiality.

The right to privacy, then, encompasses two distinct dimensions: first, the right to make certain personal decisions free from outside interference, and second, the right to control the dissemination of information about those decisions, including information set down in records, as, for example, a medical chart.[5] The former right is commonly referred to as "personal privacy," and the latter as "informational privacy." As we have already stated, the two are not necessarily coextensive. A minor, or an adult, may have the right to consent to a particular health service but not have absolute control over any record of that service which may result.

For example, a person with a venereal disease may freely consent to treatment but also may be reported to public health authorities regardless of his or her wishes.[6] So, too, for persons afflicted with certain statutorily enumerated diseases, or someone who may have been the victim of a crime; for example, a person with a gunshot wound.[7] A mother may have the right to consent to health care for her child, but if child abuse is the suspected cause of the child's health problem, she may not prevent a doctor from notifying the proper authorities.[8] Similarly, a person has the right to seek out and obtain mental health treatment, but may lose control over the records which result if the intent to injure a third person is revealed during the course of treatment.[9] Each of these examples reflects the policy judgment that the benefits which will inure to society as a result of disclosure outweigh any potential harm to the individual.

Moreover, certain practical considerations may impinge upon informational privacy rights. For example, recipients of medical services lose much control over their medical records when reimbursement claims are made to third-party payors such as insurance companies or Medicaid. Indeed such privacy considerations lead some individuals to pay out of pocket for particularly sensitive and potentially compromising health services, such as mental health services, rather than submit such claims to third-party payors and risk possible discrimination at some later time.

Thus, many states permit minors to consent to a wide range of medical services but also allow (but do not obligate) the health service provider to notify a minor's parents of such services if believed to be in the minor's best interests.[10] A few states, however, do have explicit notification requirements under certain circumstances,[11] while others, at times, forbid notification.[12]

When notification is required, permitted, or forbidden for a particular health service, this is noted in the state-by-state table. When a particular statute is silent, the normal physician–patient privilege should prevail and parental notification should not occur without the minor's consent unless there are substantial reasons for breaching confidentiality: when, for example, the already endangered life or health of the minor will be further endangered if parental notification is withheld, as in cases of suicidal ideation, or when the minor is afflicted with a life-threatening condition for which he or she refuses treatment. We realize that there may be some situations in which the minor receives truncated or inconsistent health care, perhaps because one physician is unaware of the actions of the other. We do not, however, view this factor alone as sufficient to deny confidentiality and require parental notification.

The problem of patients making only partial disclosures of medical histories applies equally to adults and minors and must be addressed in a similar manner in both instances. Thus, for example, the physician, before prescribing a medication which could cause potential negative side-effects if combined with another, must always discuss this factor with the patient; it is a basic requirement of informed consent. If the minor is accompanied by a parent, and the situation is potentially compromising, inquiries should be made in the parent's absence. If the law presumes a minor mature enough to consent to medical treatment, as it so often does, it also, by definition, presumes that the minor has sufficiently sound judgment to make adequate disclosures of his or her medical history, or to use medication as prescribed.

CHAPTER 2

Law According to Patient Status

THE LAW REGULATING the competency of minors to consent or otherwise to receive health care without parental consent can be divided into three broad categories: (1) the law based on the status of the minor; (2) the law based on the presenting health need; and (3) the law applicable for specialized situations, including, for example, minors as donors or research subjects. In this section we consider the law based on the status of the minor.

We have organized this section into eight subcategories, which, collectively, cover nearly every type of minor the health professional may encounter. We begin by discussing the minor accompanied by an adult: a parent, some other adult such as a teacher or relative, a foster parent, or institutional representative of a boarding school, camp, and the like.

We then turn to minors unaccompanied by adults, seeking health care solely on their own consent; here we discuss emancipated minors, runaway and homeless minors, college students, minors who are parents, and, in conclusion, mature minors.

These subparts, which give a general analysis of the law according to patient status, should be read in conjunction with the table at the end of the book, giving the specifics of the law as it exists in each state. We also urge the reader to refer to sections on the law according to presenting health need, or the law applicable for special situations. There are many situations in which the nature of the presenting health need, rather than the minor's status, determines the issue of who other than parents can consent.

Minors Accompanied by Adults

Minors Accompanied by a Parent

Because parents are constitutionally vested with custody and control over their minor children, they may consent to nearly every form of health care for a minor child. The consent of only one parent is sufficient unless the health professional knows or has good reason to believe that the other parent would object. In such a case the health professional, although not legally required to do so, should seek to mediate the dispute between the parents in a manner that addresses the best interests of the child. Where mediation simply is not possible and the child's welfare is threatened by delaying treatment, the provider may consider reporting the case as one of child abuse (see "Parental Refusal of Treatment" in chapter 4), seeking a court order authorizing treatment, or advising the parent favoring treatment to seek such an order, especially if the treatment is of a controversial nature or poses serious risk.[1]

Courts do not see themselves as the best forum to resolve such intrafamily disputes and try to avoid involvement in them. They generally encourage parents to reach a settlement and avoid the need for a trial. If forced to decide, a court may solicit the views of the minor if he or she is old enough to articulate them, although these views alone would not necessarily determine the court's decision. This depends not only on the views of the minor, but also the risks of the treatment, whether the treatment is supported by rational medical judgment, and whether the treatment is for the minor's benefit.

When parents are separated or divorced, the one who has actual physical control of the minor child at the time a health need arises, even if he or she is not the legal custodian, generally may give effective consent. Such may be the case if a child becomes ill during visitation, or if legal custody is jointly shared. The treating professional need not insist on proof of the accompanying parent's custodial status and may proceed in good-faith reliance on the representation of the parent, especially if treatment is of a routine nature. If the treatment is more than routine, or purely elective, the professional may want to inquire about the status and whereabouts of the other parent, seeking the consent of that parent as well if he or she possesses legal custodial rights. Treatment, however, may proceed on the physician's good faith acceptance of the representations of the presenting parent.

If there is reason to believe that such an absent parent would object to the treatment, the professional may want to seek judicial guidance. Although we did not find a case where a physician was held liable for failure to do so, this will assure that the physician does not become embroiled in a custody dispute which is ancillary to the health need of the minor. Also, if the professional has reason to question the legal authority of the accompanying parent to consent (for example, if the child may have been "kidnapped" from the custodial parent), treatment should not proceed without both parents' consent or judicial authorization, unless the presenting health need is an emergency. (See "Emergency, Urgent, and/or Necessary Health Care" in chapter 3.)

There are, however, five general situations in which the consent of one or even both parents may not be effective. These situations are addressed at greater length in succeeding sections of the book and mentioned here simply to alert the reader. First, as a general matter, parents may not consent to the sterilization of a minor child without a court order. (See "Contraception and Sterilization" in chapter 3.) Second, some states may require a court order before permitting a parent to consent to an abortion for a mentally or emotionally incompetent daughter. (See "Abortion" in chapter 3.) Third, parents cannot consent to a child's serving as an organ donor without a court order. (See "Organ Donation" in chapter 4.) Fourth, some states limit the right of the father of an illegitimate child to consent to his child's health care. (See "Minor Parents" later in this chapter.) Last, special consent is sometimes required when a child is to serve as a research subject. (See "Minors as Research Subjects" in chapter 4.)

We have treated disagreements between parent and child regarding medical treatment as a separate matter. Disagreements regarding mental health treatment (See "Mental Health Care" in chapter 3), organ donation, serving as a research subject, sterilization, contraceptive services, and abortions are each addressed in their particular sections. Other disagreements regarding medical care are discussed in the section entitled "Parent–Child Conflict" in chapter 4.

Minors Accompanied by Adults Other than Parents

Are any adults besides parents allowed to consent for the care of a minor child? What about adult relatives? What about another adult with a significant relationship to a minor such as a housekeeper, a teacher, or a community youth worker? Does the nature of the minor's health need have any bearing, as in elective cosmetic surgery versus needed treatment for an illness? Before answering these questions, consider the following situations. Cases 1, 2, and 3 are actual court cases; case 4 is hypothetical. We give the circumstances here and show how the cases were (or could have been) decided at the end of this section.

Case 1 (Actual Case)

Eleven-year-old Imogene usually lived with her parents but was temporarily in the care of an adult sister, Clara, who lived sixty miles away. Clara, a graduate nurse, suspected that Imogene had enlarged adenoids which should be removed and took the girl to a local physician who concurred and scheduled surgery. The symptoms were chronic and did not require emergency treatment, but the physician operated on Clara's consent alone and without consulting Imogene's parents. Postoperatively, Imogene died before coming out of anesthesia. Her parents sued the doctor for malpractice and for failing to obtain their consent.[1]

Case 2 (Actual Case)

Stephen, a seventeen-year-old youth residing in a community with limited medical facilities, had a rather large but benign tumor on his left ear. His local physician attempted to manage it nonsurgically, but without success. Stephen traveled alone to a neighboring city for further treatment, staying with two adult sisters and an aunt. These relatives took him to another physician, who recommended removal. Stephen entered surgery without parental consent, but apparently had consulted with his father over the telephone beforehand. Stephen died while anesthesia was being induced. The physician was sued for malpractice and operating on a minor without first obtaining parental consent.[2]

Case 3 (Actual Case)

John, a fifteen-year-old, was persuaded by his aunt to be a skin graft donor for his cousin, who had been severely burned in an accident. John's mother was ill at the time and knew nothing of the operations, which consisted of taking a tube of flesh from the skin between his axilla and waist and attaching this to his cousin. The procedure was unsuccessful, and, John, having lost a considerable amount of blood, consequently required transfusions. The physician was sued for negligence and failure to obtain the consent of John's mother.[3]

Case 4 (Hypothetical)

Nine-year-old Thomas had a large and ugly scar on his face from an earlier accident. While this presented no immediate danger, it was seriously disfiguring. Thomas's schoolmates made him the frequent butt of many cruel jokes and he became increasingly miserable and depressed. The boy desperately wanted cosmetic repair, but his parents were wholly preoccupied with their own serious marital problems and repeatedly put their son's needs aside. Thomas begged his teacher for help and she took him to a physician in hopes that something could be done. Should the physician provide treatment under these circumstances?

Historically, these cases would all have been decided one way. Except in emergency circumstances, no one other than parents were authorized to consent to the health care of a minor. Under the doctrine of parental sovereignty, parental decisions regarding a minor child, including matters of health, were deemed final and beyond the review of the state or other concerned individuals. It did not matter that some other adult seeking to represent a child was a well-intentioned close relative, friend, or neighbor, or that treatment would be in the minor's best interests. The right to consent for a child was simply a matter of authority and this was vested in parents (or legal guardians) alone. This position served two primary values. First, the minor was presumably assured mature and concerned counsel. Second, and more importantly, the right of parents to raise children as they see fit, free from outside interference, was protected.

As we stated earlier and will show throughout this book, the doctrine of parental sovereignty and privacy, while still of central importance, frequently is overruled by other overriding societal judgments. State involvement in family affairs has increased steadily over the past 150 years. Under the doctrine of *parens patriae*, which endows the state with sovereign power of guardianship over disabled and immature persons unable to manage their own affairs, the state has assumed the role of all children's ultimate protector. Society has accorded the state the right to step in and take over from parents when the latter fail to meet certain standards. (See "Historical Perspective: Parent–Child Relationships" in chapter 1.)

Despite these incursions into the doctrine of parental sovereignty, which set the rights of minor children apart from those of their parents in a number of significant ways, there has been little attention paid to whether persons other than parents (excluding representatives of the state acting as *parens patriae*) may consent to treatment of children. Specifically, there has been only limited movement toward permitting nonparental adults to consent for a minor's health care. Only a few states have such provisions[4] (which are set forth in the state-by-state table at the end of the book). Generally these laws do permit any adult who is caring for the child at the time health care is needed to act *in loco parentis* if parents are absent and/or cannot be reached; often this is within the context of emergency care.

But even in states which have no such statutes, a health professional may be found blameless for treating a minor on the consent of another adult. Thus, we cannot make a blanket statement that a health professional should never treat on the consent of a nonparental adult alone. The best we can do is to review the factors which courts have considered when such cases have come before them. In general, when the minor is mature enough to consent to treatment and the treatment is beneficial, most courts will be reluctant to hold the health professional liable. Although parental consent ordinarily would be required, decisions are often based on what seems reasonable under the particular circumstances of the case, rather than on the presence or absence of a permissory statute.

The court rulings in cases 1, 2, and 3 are illustrative. In case 1, the physician who removed the adenoids of a minor on the consent of an adult sister was found to have acted improperly. The court pointed out that there was no emergency, that the minor was quite immature, and that the adult sister had no legal custodial standing. Under the circumstances, there simply were no countervailing reasons why the requirement of parental consent should not have been observed.[5]

In case 3, where a fifteen-year-old was permitted to serve as a donor for a skin graft on the consent of his aunt, the physician was also found to have acted improperly. The court focused on two factors: the medical treatment was not for the benefit of the minor, and the minor was not sufficiently mature to give informed consent in this instance.[6] Indeed, when a minor is to serve as a donor, the consent of even the parents is probably insufficient, and the physician should obtain judicial authorization before the procedure may go forward. (See "Organ Donation" in chapter 4.)

In case 2, however, where the seventeen-year-old had a benign tumor removed from his left ear, the court ruled that actual parental consent was not required for the following reasons: the minor was near adulthood; he was accompanied by adult relatives; and he had apparently consulted with his father prior to the operation and there was no reason to believe that the father would have refused consent. The need underlying the parental consent requirement would not have been served by rigid application in this case.[7]

In our view, exonerating circumstances, as in this latter case, would not apply in the hypothetical instance of the nine-year-old boy taken by a teacher to a doctor's office for cosmetic surgery. No emergency existed, even in its broadest sense. A nine-year-old is unlikely to be sufficiently mature to give informed consent and the teacher did not have any arguable legal authority to consent on the boy's behalf; she was not even related. A health professional treating a minor under these or similar circumstances does so at the risk of liability.

But the professional is not without opportunities to help resolve such heart wrenching situations. First, and most obviously, the parents should be contacted and the seriousness of their child's disability brought to their attention. They simply may not have understood the gravity of the problem. Second, assuming that persuasion is not effective, the parents' refusal to consent can be viewed as constituting medical neglect, in which case the physician has a duty to report the case to the local child protection agency. Because Thomas clearly was adversely affected by the scar—he could not function effectively in school—it is conceivable that a court would order treatment. (For a more exhaustive discussion, see "Parental Refusal of Treatment" in chapter 4.)

It should be noted that none of these cases dealt with a health need that could possibly be construed as an emergency. That particular issue was not at question here. Broad exceptions to parental consent requirements exist in acute situations, as reviewed in detail under "Emergency, Urgent, and/or Necessary Health

Care" in chapter 3. Briefly, emergency treatment commonly is permitted without the consent of any adult; in some states the consent of a nonparental adult acting temporarily *in loco parentis* is sufficient. The definition of an emergency usually is broadly drawn, and the physician is accorded much discretion and permitted to perform a wide range of services. In addition, laws permitting minor adolescents to consent to their own care may also apply.

In conclusion, except in emergency cases, there is scant basis for permitting an adult other than the parent to consent for the health care of a minor unless there is a specific state statute allowing for such consent. Thus the provider is cautioned to proceed only where there is such a statute, or where the facts of the situation are compelling, as in case 2 or an emergency.

Minors in Foster Care

Children in foster care are those who reside outside of their natural parents' home, placed there through the auspices of the state or local government, or their designated agents. Such a residence may be in an institution, a group home, with some unrelated family, or even with a relative. By foster care we do not mean unofficial placements effected by the natural parents themselves, as, for example, a mother leaving her child with the child's grandmother. Consent issues for minors in informal placements of this nature are covered by the rules of law pertaining to minors accompanied by nonparental adults discussed earlier.

Children in foster care present special and variable considerations, depending on the nature of the placement. Placement may be initiated by a parent when, for one or another reason, the parent is unable to care for the child. This type of placement is commonly referred to as voluntary placement and may be necessary when the parent is ill or incapable of caring for the child. Voluntary placement is usually viewed as a temporary measure limited to the duration of parental incapacity.

The term "voluntary placement' however, can be misleading. If the parents do not take what the child-care agency deems to be adequate steps to regain the child from placement within a reasonable time or fail to continue to indicate their intent to take such steps, a child-care agency may attempt to terminate the parents' rights. Under these circumstances, parents who agreed to a "voluntary placement," later may find themselves faced with a court proceeding to determine whether their custodial rights should be terminated and the child freed for adoption.

Children also may be placed in foster care by parents who wish to surrender all of their rights in the child, freeing him or her for adoption. The surrender may be executed in a family, juvenile, or probate court, or by contracts outside of the court. When the surrender is validly executed, the parents lose all legal rights in and responsibility for the child and the child is in foster care pending adoption. This contrasts with voluntary placement, in which case parents retain many rights.

A third foster care process is initiated by an authorized agency, either a governmental entity or its agent (e.g., a child-protective agency) acting without the parents' consent. Involuntary removal most commonly occurs when a parent is alleged to have abused or neglected a child. The child is removed from the parental home for his or her protection while the fitness of the parents to retain custody is evaluated. If the child is to be permanently removed from the care of natural parents, a court proceeding is necessary. (Current policy, however, seeks family reunion and the provision of external supports to strengthen parental competency when the child is in foster care against parental will.)

When a child is in foster care, the parents retain many rights over his or her medical treatment as long as their right to custody has not been terminated or they have not surrendered the child for adoption. Statutes which address this specific question generally permit custodial institutions or foster parents to consent to medical care for the child which is ordinary, routine, or necessary. Even in the absence of a statute, this would most likely be true; otherwise, there might be no one to consent for a child's day-to-day medical needs.

On the other hand, if the treatment is major, risky, or elective, the natural parents, not the foster care authority, probably retain the residuary legal right to consent. But all considerations of who has authority to consent in foster care situations are of secondary concern when an emergency exists. In this situation, emergency principles apply.

When the rights of parents have been terminated by court action, or the child has been surrendered for adoption, the state is, in effect, the legal guardian and generally delegates to a representative of the foster care agency the authority to consent to both routine necessary care and major or elective health care.

While many states have statutes regarding foster care, few specifically address the issue of medical consent. However, the state agency responsible for foster care should be able to advise on applicable administrative guidelines and regulations. In the absence of such advice, it is fair to say that the individual caretaker accompanying a foster child in need of medical treatment is generally aware of who must provide legal consent. If this individual is not aware, the supervising social service agency assuredly will be conversant in the local rules and should be consulted.

Finally, the state as the guardian for a minor does not hold greater rights over the minor than would the natural parents. The principles discussed throughout this book apply to minors in foster care in exactly the same way as they do to those who live at home. Minors in foster care may for example become emancipated, may be considered mature minors, may consent to VD and sex-related health care, may obtain contraceptives, and in general may enjoy the same rights as other minors.

Foster Care: Summary

1. Foster parents or representatives of custodial institutions generally may consent to routine or necessary care of the minor they are responsible for on a day-to-day basis.
2. If the proposed treatment is elective, major, or bears significant risks, and placement has occurred as a result of voluntary action on the part of the natural parents, the consent of the natural parents should be obtained. If their whereabouts are unknown, the supervising social service agency should be contacted.
3. If the proposed treatment is elective, major, or bears significant risks, and placement was initiated by a governmental entity, and parental rights have been terminated, or the minor surrendered for adoption, the supervising social services agency may consent.
4. If the health need is an emergency, general emergency principles govern. (See chapter 3.)
5. Laws permitting minors to consent without parental consent apply as much to those in foster care as to those residing with natural parents.

Minors in Detention Facilities

When a minor is in a detention facility, the parents retain the right to consent to the minor's health care except for routine day-to-day treatment. If the treatment is elective, complex, or high-risk, the natural parents' consent should be obtained.

Minors in Boarding Schools, Camps, and Related Institutions

Laws governing minors who are temporarily living away from home at schools (with the exception of colleges; see "Other Minors Away from Home" in a later section of this chapter), camps, or other such institutions are no different from those for minors living at home. Such minors do not acquire any emancipating rights; they are not self-supporting or managing their own financial affairs, and their supervising personnel do not have any greater authority to consent than do other nonparental adults accompanying a child. When searching for authority of a school or camp to treat a minor without parental consent, reference should be made to sections of chapter 3 dealing with specific health needs such as emergency care, sex-related services, or substance abuse treatment; or to the following sections of this chapter, which deal with such aspects of the patient's status as parenthood, marriage, maturity, and age of consent. If parental consent is required for the treatment, the parents should be contacted and their consent obtained. The institution should not be seen as standing in the stead of the parents unless there is a specific law to the contrary.

It is common practice for such institutions to have obtained a written blanket consent from parents prior to their children's enrollment. This is as valid as any blanket consent and may be honored accordingly. It is generally satisfactory for ordinary, low-risk, and noninvasive care. A separate parental consent should be obtained for invasive treatment or that which incurs significant risks. No consent is necessary when emergency care is involved.[1]

Minors Unaccompanied by Adults

Age of Consent

Historically, the age of majority was twenty-one. After the voting age for federal elections was constitutionally lowered to eighteen in 1971, nearly every state followed suit by lowering its own age of majority accordingly.[1] But we make a mistake if we think that there is a single age at which a person becomes an adult for all purposes. While every state has a statute providing for a general age of majority, each also has a number of exceptions according minors adult rights or responsibilities for specific and limited purposes, reflecting the policy judgment that under certain circumstances, minors should be permitted to function as adults even before the age of majority out of capacity or pragmatic need. The converse is also true; some persons above the age of majority have limitations impressed on them in relation to certain privileges accorded to most adults.

New York State, for example, has set the general age of majority at eighteen,[2] but a female is no longer entitled to statutory rape protections and is deemed "old enough" to enter into sexual relations at age seventeen.[3] On the other hand, an individual of eighteen years, a legal adult, may not purchase or consume alcoholic beverages until age twenty-one because of the association between automotive accidents and intoxicated young drivers.[4] In another example, sixteen-year-olds are presumed to be "infants" at law for almost all purposes, but if they are charged with crimes their cases will be adjudicated by adult criminal courts rather than juvenile courts, the reason being punitive rather than rehabilitative intent. Children as young as thirteen, when charged with very serious crimes, may be punished as adults.[5] And, at the opposite end of the scale, although eighteen-year-olds are considered adults for almost all purposes, they are still deemed to be financially dependent upon their parents until age twenty-one, and parents may be required to contribute toward the support of their children between ages eighteen and twenty who apply for public assistance.[6] Similar exceptions to the general age of majority, both upward and downward, exist in every state. In all cases, however, a person who has reached the age of majority may consent to his or her own health care.

Furthermore, many of the downward exceptions specifically apply to young people who seek medical care. Indeed, these exceptions are so extensive that the general requirement of parental consent has been nearly obliterated for older adolescents. The underlying policy judgment is that the benefit of teenage minors' independent access to medical care far outweighs any advantage gained by requiring parental consent, which could deter the young person from obtaining timely treatment. Several states even have rather sweeping statutes which explicitly permit minors to consent to all forms of health care, even though they are not legal adults.[7] Thus the age of majority of a particular state does not provide a clear line indicating that those below that age may not consent to treatment. Each situation must be examined independently. A minor who seeks treatment for drug abuse is, in the eyes of the law, different from a minor who seeks cosmetic surgery; so, too, a seventeen-year-old who lives away from home permanently is viewed differently than a thirteen-year-old still living with his or her family. These differences are reflected in many of the state statutes, as well as in case law.

In the state-by-state table, with the exception of several states, we have listed statutes which set forth the general age of majority for that state. Minors who have attained this age may indisputably consent to health care. In states where minors are permitted to consent to all forms of health care before reaching the age of majority, we have set forth the specific enabling statute, rather than the general age of majority statute. It should be noted that these latter statutes only apply to the age at which the minor may consent to medical care and not to any other sphere. The reader should be sure to review other sections of the book to ascertain whether a minor may consent to care even though a health-care–specific or general age of majority statute is not helpful.

Emancipated Minors

Emancipation concepts have derived more from case law than statutory law; state legislatures have only recently begun to look at this issue. Based on an analysis of what the courts have said, it is clear that emancipated minors indeed can obtain health services on their own. We have been unable to discover a single instance of a physician's being found liable for providing care to an emancipated youth on his or her own consent and without the consent of parents. Indeed, in one of the few recent cases which address this particular point, *Smith* v. *Seibly*,[1] the court ruled that the minor was competent to consent.

In *Smith*, a married minor, who was no longer under his parents' control nor dependent on them for financial support and functioned as the head of his own family, suffered from myasthenia gravis. He and his wife decided he should have a vasectomy to limit the size of his family. He signed a consent form and the surgical procedure took place. The minor later sought to disaffirm his consent because of legal incapacity. The jury found the minor emancipated and thus able to give consent. The jury's decision was upheld on appeal.

Despite the well-established nature of the emancipation doctrine, health care providers have been reluctant to accept it. Confusion about the criteria by which emancipation is determined, concern about possible liability if an incorrect determination is made, and doubts about who is financially responsible have combined to sap this doctrine of its vitality and authority as a basis for providing treatment. Nonetheless, clear directions can be gleaned from the substantial body of case law that does exist. In addition, an increasing number of states are now enacting relevant statutes which provide additional clarification and support.

Confusion regarding the emancipation doctrine stems partly from the evolution of the concept. Initially, a minor was emancipated when his parents relinquished their claims on his earnings.[2] Over time, emancipation came to mean parental relinquishment of control over the child's behavior and personal affairs. Emancipation was conveyed by the parents' affirmative surrender of their nurturant and protective role. The *definition* of emancipation, however, was not substantively changed; a minor still had to be living apart from parents with their permission and earning his or her own support through traditional employment, although minors living at home and retaining their own earnings could be considered emancipated in certain circumstances.[3] Also, married minors and minors in the armed services were considered emancipated. By implication, emancipated youths also had to be above the age of compulsory school attendance. Not only were those of lesser years expected to be in the classroom, but the ability to be self-supporting was severely limited by statutory restrictions on the nature of their employment and the number of hours they could work.

In the past two decades, however, the emancipation doctrine has changed not only its derivative base but also its definition. In parallel with emerging concepts of minors' rights and the mature minor doctrine, young people themselves now have some determining force. Parental relinquishment of claims to supervisory and controlling rights may now occur as much by passive default or simple incapacity as by affirmative and deliberate permission.

Moreover, the ability of a minor to function as a self-supporting individual need not be demonstrated by traditional employment alone. Today the general definition of an emancipated minor is one who (1) is living separate and apart from parents with or *without* their consent; (2) is self-supporting but *without regard to the source of income*; and (3) is managing his or her own financial affairs.[4] Further, as before, a married minor or a minor in the armed services is considered emancipated, and it is possible for a minor living at home, paying room and board, and making his or her own decisions to establish emancipation.

The departure of a minor from his or her family no longer requires affirmative parental action and can be carried out on the minor's initiative alone.[5] Simply the failure of a parent to take effective steps in compelling the minor to return home is sufficient to comply with this particular criterion. The minor need only have established a separate and independent residence. This may be next door to the parental home or in some other state; the minor may live in a single room with some other family or rent his or her own apartment. This arrangement, however, must be a deliberate and permanent step, at least by intention. An impulsive runaway gesture in which the minor expects ultimately to return home does not meet the requirement. Some of the newer emancipation statutes specifically address this point by requiring the lapse of a certain period of time before a separate residence can be deemed established.

Second, while the ability to be self-supporting has long been a critical element of the emancipation definition, this criterion no longer must be met only through legitimate employment. Indeed, the source of the minor's income is irrelevant.[6] It need not even be a legal or morally uplifting source. Nor need the income be earned; living on loans or an inheritance or monetary gifts qualifies equally as well.

Finally, management of one's own financial affairs simply requires that the minor provide for his or her own food, clothing, and shelter; pay his or her own bills; and handle his or her own money rather than turning it over to someone else. The minor's credit rating, however, is not at issue. (As discussed earlier in this chapter, minors in boarding schools or in various other institutional residences, with the exception of colleges, customarily do not manage their own finances as defined above and would not qualify as emancipated.)

Note, however, that minors who are living at home but working and contributing to the family's support also may be considered emancipated if, in addition, they make most of their own decisions, manage most of their own personal affairs, and take care of their personal expenses.[7]

There also are variations on the emancipation doctrine in which the particular status of a minor by definition makes him or her emancipated and requires no further qualification. Thus minors in the armed services or minors who are or have been married[8] are emancipated. Minors who are parents are emancipated without regard to age, residence, finances, or other factors. (See "Minor Parents" later in this chapter.) In some states, simply being a high school graduate is sufficient to emancipate for purposes of consenting to health care.[9]

Given these emancipation concepts, how may they be applied in the health care situation? What documentation is required? How should the question of parental notification be resolved? And who is responsible for payment? We will answer each of these questions by posing some hypothetical situations as a framework for subsequent discussion.

Documentation and Misrepresentations: Case 1 (Hypothetical)

Shirley, age sixteen, went to a physician specializing in weight loss through hypnotherapy. She was somewhat chubby, had tried many other methods to no avail, and very much wanted to lose fifteen pounds. When asked about parental permission, Shirley stated she was a high school graduate, had been living away from home for the past six months, was supporting herself as a grocery store checkout clerk, and therefore was emancipated. She also had the cash in hand to pay. There was no reason to doubt her representations, and, accordingly, she was treated on her own consent. But, in truth, Shirley was not emancipated. She still was a high school student living at home and supported by her parents. She had misrepresented her status because her parents did not approve of hypnotherapy and had refused to take her to the doctor themselves. She had taken the money to pay out of her college savings account.

Documentation and Misrepresentation: Case 2 (Hypothetical)

Diane, age fourteen, visited a physician on her own to obtain a physical examination as required by the job she soon was to start. She explained that she no longer lived at home and considered herself to be emancipated. The physician was quite surprised, because unbeknownst to Diane, he had met her parents at a social gathering only two weeks before. They had told him of their problems with their headstrong daughter, who was more interested in obtaining money to buy clothes than in improving her poor academic performance. They further spoke of their opposition to her wish to work after school instead of attending to her studies. Thus the physician was well aware that Diane had been living at home and supported by her parents only two weeks before. When further questioned about her status, Diane only responded in vague and elusive terms. The physician also found Diane to be quite immature.

These two situations raise the question of misrepresentation. Both patients allege that they are emancipated and entitled to consent. If their statements were true, both indeed would qualify. But in fact, Shirley and Diane are still unemancipated. The significant difference is that there is nothing to repudiate Shirley's statements; they seem honest and plausible. On the other hand, the physician had personal knowledge raising considerable suspicion about Diane's veracity.

The representations of a minor may be taken at face value as long as they seem reasonable and sincere, and as long as the provider has no reason to doubt them and acts accordingly in good faith. Definitive documentation is not required, only appropriate assessment and professional judgment. Thus Shirley may be treated on her own consent without fear of liability. But if, as in Diane's case, facts are known or suspected that negate what the minor says, or if the minor's alleged status seems implausible, additional investigation is indicated. Diane should not be treated as an emancipated minor without further clarification.

Parental Notification (Hypothetical)

Sixteen-year-old Mary was brought to a hospital clinic by friends who were concerned about her loss of weight. She had run away from home in another state six months before because of abusive and alcoholic parents. Since that time she had not communicated with her parents at all and had lived in her friends' apartment; she was self-supporting but through undisclosed means, and managed her own financial affairs. There was some suspicion that she may have been prostituting herself. Medical evaluation determined that Mary was suffering from anorexia nervosa, although major weight loss had not yet occurred and she was in no present medical danger. Despite the potential seriousness of her condition, Mary refused to have her parents notified.

Mary definitely is emancipated under newer definitions and quite capable of consenting to her own health care, but the nature of her condition is such that professional judgment might well deem parental advisement appropriate even if Mary does not agree. Many states which have statutes allowing emancipated minors to consent to medical care also allow health services providers to notify parents if the situation warrants it.[10] It is important to note, however, that no statutes *require* notification and a few even limit the circumstances in which this may take place. In Massachusetts, parents may not be notified unless life or limb is endangered. Minnesota allows notification only when the failure to do so would seriously jeopardize the minor's health.

In states without statutes, the general rule of thumb is that notification is never required, but parents may be advised if the physician, in exercising professional judgment, believes their involvement important to the minor's health, broadly defined. The degree of seriousness is a contributing factor. Mary's present condition does not warrant parental notification against her will; she is in no immediate medical danger, and establishing a trusting therapeutic relationship is more important than alienating her by disregarding her request for confidentiality. Should her condition deteriorate, however, the physician would be justified in notifying Mary's parents if he or she deemed this important to her care—a matter of some debate in light of her family's history. Parental notification simply to avoid the possibility of provoking parental litigation is an insufficient reason and could well be cause for the emancipated minor to launch his or her own claims of breach of privacy.

Payment Issues (Hypothetical)

Frank, a seventeen-year-old army private, and Ann, his sixteen-year-old wife, went to a physician's office because they both had been experiencing mild diarrhea following a camping trip in the mountains several weeks before. Frank produced both his army identification and marriage certificate documenting their emancipation. The doctor saw Frank and Ann for a total of three visits each, performed stool examinations on them both (revealing giardiasis), and dispensed appropriate medication for a total cost of $200. After failing to respond to a number of the physician's bills, which had been put in the hands of a collection agency, Frank finally called to say that he just had been discharged from the army, had not yet gotten a job, and had no money to pay. He suggested that since he and his wife were still both minors, either his or her parents should be billed instead.

The liability of a parent for services rendered to an emancipated minor is an often-litigated issue. While the courts have not been unanimous in their resolution of claims, most decisions have ruled that parents cannot be compelled to pay for services sought out and consented to by an emancipated minor unless they, the parents, have specifically accepted financial responsibility. We believe this would probably be the case even if an unemancipated minor has misrepresented his or her status. The doctrine of emancipation clearly involves personal financial responsibility as well as an independent living situation. Thus the ability of an emancipated minor to consent to health care also involves the responsibility to pay. In all likelihood, the physician would not be successful in suing the parents of Frank and Ann for payment. (See "The Payment Question" at the end of chapter 6.)

In summary, a few points are central. An increasing number of states are enacting statutes which allow minors to appeal to the courts for a declaration of emancipation for many purposes. To qualify, such youths usually must have lived apart from their families for a reasonable period of time; they must usually be self-supporting and managing their own financial affairs; and they must usually give other evidence of being able to function in an independent manner. While we have noted those states having such laws in the statutory references table, we have not detailed their requirements, as this is a court, not health provider, determination. We would hold, however, that minors in these states need *not* have received such a declaration in order to be considered emancipated for health care purposes alone. They may be assessed according to the general principles we have already defined.

Second, minor parents are considered emancipated for the purposes of health care for themselves and their children. We have not included this topic here because parenthood has a range of additional concerns and is addressed in its own section later in this chapter. We refer the reader accordingly. As we have already noted, other life-status situations which can be considered emancipating in almost every case, even when not addressed by statute, include married minors and minors serving in the armed forces.

Third, there usually will be some other basis for treatment on their own consent for those minors who are functioning in a relatively self-directed manner but do not clearly qualify as emancipated. Statutes conveying a specific age of majority for health care purposes and mature-minor statutes also apply. In addition, laws pertaining to the nature of the health need should be looked to for alternative support, including those relating to substance abuse, sex-related health care, and emergencies.

Fourth, emancipation may convey only the capacity to consent for *beneficial* treatment: that is, treatment directly intended to prevent or remediate a health need of the minor himself or herself. This would not include blood or tissue donation for the benefit of another. Eligibility to consent to blood donation usually is defined by age in specific statutes. We refer the reader to the detailed discussion on research and organ donation rules to be found in chapter 4.

Finally, it is implicit that any consent given by an emancipated youth should be informed and that he or she should have the capacity to give an informed consent. This should not pose a significant problem with respect to health care, in that any minor who is sufficiently competent as to be functionally emancipated should also be sufficiently mature to have that capacity.

Married minors. Minors who are or have been married are considered emancipated for the purposes of health care without further requirements including a residence of their own. Many states have specific enabling statutory provisions. But even in the absence of such a law, treatment may proceed on the consent of a minor who is now or ever has been married. Further, this may be done on the good-faith reliance of the health professional on the minor's representations, and documentation is not required; the same principles apply here as for other youths alleging emancipation.

Other Minors Away from Home

A minor may be away from home and yet not fit within the classic definition of an emancipated minor, and there may not be specific laws or court decisions permitting the minor to consent to medical treatment without parental consent. In this section we address such situations.

Runaway and homeless youth. Young people are running away from home in ever-increasing numbers. One recent survey estimates that 733,000 young people leave home annually without parental consent.[1] There is little to indicate a reversal of this trend. Therefore, the health professional may be frequently asked to provide services to young people who may not fit within the definition of emancipation due to the fact that they may have only recently departed from the parental home and not clearly established a separate residence.

The fact that a minor has run away from home does not, in and of itself, convey the capacity to consent to health care. Other sources of authority may need to be found. The nature of the need, the mature-minor doctrine, and, possibly, new definitions of emancipation may apply if the young person has indeed permanently established a separate residence—although frequently this is not the case. Once the minor's health problem and personal status have been identified, the practitioner should consult the relevant sections of chapter 3, "Law According to Patient Need," and, in this chapter, the earlier section "Emancipated Minors," as well as a subsequent section, "Mature Minors."

Health providers will most frequently encounter runaway youths when they are in need of emergency or necessary health services. Of course, normal emergency considerations will apply. But the range of health services that may be provided under the name "emergency" may be broader for runaways than for others. As noted by Angela Holder, author of *Legal Issues in Pediatrics and Adolescent Medicine*:

> As a practical matter, however, any court would undoubtedly hold that a runaway in need of treatment who refuses to identify his parents or tell a physician how to locate them so that they may be contacted for their consent, may be presumed emancipated for purposes of consent. This would be true even if the treatment is necessary but cannot be classified as an emergency.[2]

Holder recommends that the treating facility carefully note that the minor did not agree to parental notification and refused to give the necessary information for this to occur, and then have the minor sign the statement.[3] To that we would add that the health professional should document in the chart what efforts were made in attempting to convince the minor to involve his or her parents.

Even in the absence of such documentation, the risk of liability is remote. The courts generally presume that physicians act in good faith and for the benefit of their patients. A review of scores of cases regarding treatment of minors without parental consent suggests that physicians are rarely held liable for providing needed medical care to runaways on their own consent even if for something less than an emergency.

Additional support can be found in the mature-minor doctrine. Any minor not living at home, regardless of the circumstances, who recognizes that he or she has a health need, takes the necessary steps to obtain it, and appears capable of giving an informed consent assuredly evidences considerable maturity. We find no substantive reason for not rendering health care to such a runaway minor on his or her own consent when the parents' whereabouts cannot be determined and the treatment is for the minor's benefit.

College students. Many minor college students do not fit cleanly within the definition of emancipation because, while they may live away from home, they often remain financially dependent upon their parents. Nonetheless, a parent probably could not recover damages against a physician for treating a college student without parental consent, no matter what the presenting health need. Holder notes:

> It is probably wise to attempt to notify the parent of a [minor] college student who requires a major surgical procedure or medical intervention that carries a high degree of risk but, if the physician proceeds to treat him without doing so and certainly if the college student has objected to notification of the parent, it is highly unlikely that a successful suit could be maintained by his parents.[4]

Minor Parents

Minors who are parents present special situations in terms of consenting to care for both themselves and their children. These areas, along with other aspects of reproductive health care, are not solely matters of state regulation; they also involve minors' constitutional rights.

Consent for the children. It has been widely recognized that the number of minor parents is rapidly increasing. It is also evident that someone must be able to consent to the health care of their children. Most states now statutorily grant minor parents the authority to consent to the medical care of their children in the same manner as adult parents. Social policy inclines to the view that if minor parents' rights in their children have not been terminated for particular cause, they retain all the rights and responsibilities of adults, including those pertaining to their children.

The fact that a particular state may not have an enabling statute is irrelevant, because this view is required by the United States Constitution and its repeated interpretations holding that all parents have a fundamental right as against all others to the custody and control of their offspring.[1]

Children born out of wedlock. Separate issues are raised when the child is born out of wedlock, as is common for children of minors. Few states specifically distinguish between the rights of natural mothers and fathers (either minor or adult), although natural mothers are generally presumed to have custody and the primary caretaker role. (Mississippi is an exception: its statute provides that the father of an illegitimate child may not consent to treatment of the child solely on the basis of fatherhood.[2])

Nonetheless, natural fathers do hold certain constitutional rights vis-à-vis their illegitimate offspring, although not necessarily the same as for mothers. In *Caban* v. *Mohammed,* the Supreme Court made this point quite clear.[3] The case involved a New York statute granting the mother of an illegitimate child a veto power over the child's adoption, but denying the same right to the natural father. On appeal, the Court struck down the statute on the ground that its denial of right to a father who had established a substantial relationship with his illegitimate child was unconstitutional. Statutes which treat mothers and fathers of illegitimate children differently, particularly when the father has assumed an active parental role, may be constitutionally suspect unless they can be shown to support important social policies. To date, there has not been a ruling on a statute similar to the one in Mississippi pertaining to the right of such fathers to consent to the health care of their children, and it is not possible for us to predict if it could withstand constitutional scrutiny.

When there is no applicable statute or, even if present, the statute does not distinguish between natural mothers and natural fathers of an illegitimate child, a father who presents his child for necessary, urgent, or routine treatment, but does not have legal custody, should be viewed as having the authority to consent to the child's treatment, especially where paternity has been acknowledged or established. But when the treatment is serious or risky, although not an emergency, the health provider should inquire about the whereabouts of the natural mother and the circumstances by which the father came to have possession. If it appears that both parents are acting in concert on behalf of the child, treatment may proceed on the father's consent. But if there is any implication of controversy, the mother's consent should be obtained as well. While it is not clear that this would be a legal requirement, we simply cannot ignore the fact that in the vast majority of cases, young mothers, either by default or court order, have custody of illegitimate children, and common sense dictates further inquiry. Of course, should the father have legal custody—a rare but possible circumstance—he does have the exclusive capacity to act on his child's behalf.

Last, if the health professional knows a minor father does not have authority over an illegitimate offspring, treatment for nonemergency conditions should not proceed. This could include, for example, the fact that the father's rights over the child have been terminated, or that he "kidnapped" the child from the natural mother.

Minor parents' consent for themselves. In all cases, minor parents are considered emancipated and may consent not only to the health care of their children, but to their own health care as well. The absence of a specific permissory statute is not important.

Mature Minors

The mature-minor doctrine is another evolving exception to the general requirement of parental consent to treatment of a minor. This doctrine holds that if a minor is of sufficient intelligence and maturity to understand and appreciate both the benefits and risks of the proposed medical or surgical treatment, then the minor may consent to that treatment without parental consent, other issues (including the fact that the minor is still living at home and financially dependent) notwithstanding. Most simply, mature minors differ from emancipated minors in that they are living at home, are not contributing to room and board, or are not parents themselves, married, or members of the armed forces; they are the most typical adolescents. The basis of their authority to consent derives from the developmental maturation of cognition, not from life-style status, as for emancipated minors, or age, as for those who have achieved majority.

In essence, the mature-minor doctrine simply addresses the young person's ability to give an informed consent. Neither the nature of the health need nor the minor's life-style status need be specified for application. But, as we shall detail further on, there are a number of qualifying factors, and the mature-minor doctrine does not provide authority for the treatment of all adolescents on their own consent without discrimination. However, it does offer a useful basis for providing health care to many minor youths in situations where treatment is indicated but no other exceptions apply and parental involvement is problematic.

The mature-minor doctrine, like the emancipation doctrine, was, and remains today, largely a creation of the courts with but limited statutory codification. Only five states have laws specifically permitting mature minors to consent to health care in general without parental consent. Many states, however, have more narrowly incorporated this doctrine by implication in their statutes addressing minors' consent to treatment of specified health needs such as sex-related problems and drug abuse.

The principles of the mature-minor doctrine do have significant precedent in case law and may be applied in any state. A number of courts have addressed this issue, and their decisions provide a clear basis for establishing guidelines as to how and when this doctrine may be used. We may best define these guidelines by examining some actual cases which have come before the courts.

Case 1

Shirley, age nineteen (when the age of majority was twenty-one), sought out medical treatment for a skin disorder. She consented to the performance of an operation, and a biopsy was performed. She later sued the physician, claiming that her consent was invalid because she was a minor when she gave it.[1]

Case 2

Seventeen-year-old Nancy caught her finger in a door while visiting her mother in the hospital. She sustained the traumatic amputation of a fingertip and was taken to the emergency room, where a pinch graft was applied by a resident surgeon. Nancy's mother later sued, alleging that her daughter was a minor and therefore could not consent to the operation.[2]

Case 3

Christine, age eighteen (at a time when the age of majority was twenty-one), sought out, consented to, and underwent cosmetic surgery on her nose. Apparently dissatisfied with the results, Christine later sued the physician for assault and battery, alleging that her earlier consent was not valid due to her minority.[3]

Case 4

John, age fifteen, lived with his mother. His cousin, Ruth, had been severely burned and needed a skin graft but had been unable to locate a compatible tissue donor. John's aunt persuaded him to be tested and to be the donor if he should match. This proved to be the case and John submitted to a tube graft procedure. This was not successful, and in the process John both suffered sufficient blood loss as to require a transfusion and ended up with a substantial scar. John's mother had not even been informed of the operation, much less given her consent.[4]

The minors in cases 1, 2, and 3 were all adjudged mature enough to consent to their surgical procedures without parental involvement. In Shirley's case, the court stated: "[T]here is nothing to suggest that [Shirley], at the time of executing the consent, had not reached the age of discretion,[5] or that [she] was under any physical or mental disability." Nancy was noted to be "of sufficient age and maturity to know and understand the nature and consequences of the 'pinch graft' utilized in the repair of her finger" and thereby was held capable of giving an informed consent.[6]

One of the principles which emerges from the rulings in cases 1 and 2 is that the mature-minor doctrine is primarily applicable to older youths, but without specificity as to exact age. We can, however, be quite certain that minors aged fifteen years or more would qualify. Despite a diligent search by us and other authors among reported court decisions, no decision has been found where damages were awarded against a physician for providing needed and beneficial treatment of any nature, including surgery, to a minor over the age of fifteen on the minor's own consent and without that of the parents.[7]

Nancy's case also illustrates another principle. Here the courts also found that because the medical procedures were necessary, there was no reason to believe that the parents would not have consented to the treatment had they known. Thus the mature-minor doctrine does have some conceptual overlap with rules governing emergency care. But the definition of "necessary" as employed in the mature-minor doctrine is even more relaxed than its definition in emergency care.

In some instances, the mature-minor doctrine may be applied to elective as well as necessary procedures. In case 3, involving cosmetic surgery, the court said:

> A charge that this eighteen-year-old plaintiff [when the age of majority was twenty-one] could not consent to . . . a *simple operation* would seem inconsistent with the conclusion of our General Assembly, that any female child of sixteen can prevent the taking of liberties with

> her person from being rape[d] merely by consenting thereto at the time such liberties are taken. . . . [The] performance of a surgical operation upon an eighteen-year-old girl with her consent will ordinarily not amount to an assault and battery for which damages may be recoverable even though the consent of such girl's parents or guardian has not been secured.[8]

Thus the court refused to hold the physician liable for assault and battery.

In case 4, however (also discussed earlier in this chapter, under "Minors Accompanied by Adults Other Than Parents"), treatment was neither necessary nor even for John's benefit, but was for the benefit of his cousin. Moreover, John suffered significant harm in the process. In ruling on the case, the court made a number of observations. It first noted that there was a technical requirement for parental consent deriving from common law principles relating to contracts and torts, but that this was not absolute and there were a number of permissible exceptions including maturity of the minor in question. The court, however, refused to extend the mature-minor doctrine to John's particular case or to any case in which treatment was not for the minor's own benefit. The court said: When "a surgical operation [is] not for the benefit of the person operated on but for another, and also [is] so involved in its technique as to require a mature mind to understand precisely what the donor [is] offering to give," the mature minor doctrine does not apply.[9]

The principles elucidated in this latter case give further support to the mature-minor doctrine both by simply invoking the term and by noting that there are instances when mature minors can consent to their own health care and the consent of parents is not necessary. But, clearly, this doctrine does not extend to nonbeneficial care, including tissue donation, particularly when complex issues and significant risks are involved which could be difficult for any patient to appreciate.

One can also infer from this ruling that there may be some constraints on applying the mature-minor doctrine even in beneficial situations when the contemplated procedure is singularly risky and/or involved. Unfortunately, there is no additional case law direction. All of the decisions which look at the applicability of the mature-minor doctrine in relation to beneficial care deal with relatively straightforward and easily understood procedures. But we suspect that the courts would be likely to see the involvement of a parent as important and to limit the mature-minor doctrine when the proposed treatment is of a particularly serious or complex nature, and therefore difficult to understand in full and proper measure.

Based on the foregoing and other court decisions, it is evident that the concept of the mature minor has variable applicability and depends on the assessment of a number of factors. But these are not difficult to define, and we consider the risk of liability for treating a mature minor on his or her own consent to be negligible if the following criteria are met:

1. The minor is fifteen years of age or over. (Note that this is without regard to the minor's residential or financial status.)
2. The minor is able to give an informed consent; that is, in the judgment of the treating physician, the minor appears to be of sufficient maturity and intelligence to understand and appreciate the benefits and risks of the proposed treatment and to make a reasoned decision based on such knowledge.
3. The proposed treatment is for the minor's benefit and not for the benefit of another.
4. The proposed treatment is deemed necessary according to best professional judgment. (Even with unnecessary, elective procedures whose risks are easily understood the physician is only likely to face the award of token damages at most.)
5. The treatment does not involve complex, high-risk medical procedures or complex, high-risk surgery.[10]

One question which may well be asked is just how maturity is to be assessed and what yardsticks may be applied. The courts appear to be content to simply look at the minor's age and his or her evident understanding of the benefits and risks of the treatment involved. Admittedly, these parameters lack precision, but no other measures need be applied. The courts have never required more than the treating professional's best judgment and good-faith assessment. As we have noted more than once, the courts generally presume that physicians act in an ethical manner and for their patients' best benefit and are unlikely to presume otherwise unless there is clear evidence to the contrary.

In documenting the minor's maturity, nothing more is required than a notation in the patient's chart that the minor did indeed appear to be sufficiently intelligent to understand the benefits and risks of the proposed treatment, together with a statement as to just what benefits and risks were discussed. The minor, of course, should read and sign an appropriate consent form in the same manner as would an adult.

In sum, courts which have addressed the mature-minor doctrine have employed it to work reasonable results between physician and patient. Thus, when the rigid requirement of parental consent has not served the purposes which underlie it, courts have been quite willing to discard it and apply the mature-minor doctrine.

CHAPTER 3

Law According to Patient Need

IN THE PREVIOUS CHAPTER we addressed the eligibility of minors to consent to health care on their own based on such indicators as age, life-style, and cognitive maturity. These are all markers which have little to do with the particular health problem at hand. In this chapter we shift our focus to examine the law from the perspective of the presenting complaint.

Virtually all states have statutes which permit minors afflicted with certain conditions to obtain treatment on their own and without parental consent. These include sexually transmitted diseases, pregnancy-related care, substance abuse, and mental health care. Young people engaged in parentally forbidden behaviors with significant health risks or in need of psychological assistance for highly personal matters are unlikely to seek out professional assistance in a timely manner if parental consent is a prerequisite. To most adolescents, the perceived costs of parental discovery and fear of possible retribution—or, at the least, psychological devaluation—far outweigh the costs of ignoring a health need.

Abortion and contraceptive care must be viewed differently. These are the only situations in which the minor's right to self-consent is constitutionally derived. Following on a sequence of rulings endowing minors with certain constitutional rights, the United States Supreme Court has declared that minors also have privacy rights in these two areas.

We have also included emergency care and care for the minor who is the victim of a crime in this chapter. Treatment of minors on their own is allowed in these situations because it is often presumed that if the parents were present, they would consent to the treatment.

Each of the preceding topics will be discussed in relation to the general trends in the law. Armed with this background information, the reader can then knowledgeably refer to the table of statutes for the particular state in question and the details on applicable rules. But it must not be forgotten that even in the absence of an enabling statute pertaining to a specific health need, there commonly will be some other basis, such as the minor's status, on which a minor may be treated in the absence of parental consent. Therefore, reference to other possibly relevant sections of the book is recommended.

Emergency, Urgent, and/or Necessary Health Care

Health professionals are frequently asked to provide emergency, urgent, or necessary health care to minors in the absence of parental consent. The whereabouts of the parents (for purposes of discussion, when the word "parent" is used it also includes legal guardians) may be unknown; or the whereabouts of the parents may be known, but it is not possible to contact them expeditiously. The question then arises of who, if anyone, is required to consent to the treatment of the minor. Interestingly, in such cases the fact that the patient is a minor is not really of critical importance. What if an adult patient who required urgent care were unconscious? The issue of consent is essentially the same. The physician is allowed, of course, to treat the patient according to his or her best judgment; no definitive consent is required. Consent under such circumstances is implied from the facts: that is, given the urgency of the health need, any reasonable individual would want to be treated promptly, and any reasonable parents would wish the same for their child.

Because of the frequency with which such situations occur, nearly every state has enacted specific statutes (as summarized in the statutory reference table at the end of this book) addressing the treatment of minors under emergency circumstances, and the governing rules should be relatively clear. Health service providers, however, tend to hold a variety of misconceptions which have the effect of unduly limiting the full application of statutory intent.

In clarifying these problems, we may best begin by looking at some actual cases which have come before the courts. But keep in mind that suits for assault and battery for failure to first obtain parental consent are extremely rare. In every one of the following cases the physician was sued primarily for negligence, and the issue of assault and battery for lack of parental consent was used as a secondary buttress. Such a claim is nearly always asserted in addition to claims that the physician treated the minor in a negligent manner; had there been no resultant harm, challenge over the absence of parental consent would, in all probability, never have taken place.

Case 1

Seven-year-old Helen broke her right forearm while playing in the school playground. The principal tried to reach Helen's mother by telephoning her place of employment, but without success. He did not attempt to call the mother at home or to take Helen there, although it was only a mile from her school. Instead Helen was taken to a local physician, who determined that the arm was fractured and reduction under anesthesia indicated. She died during the procedure. Helen's mother subsequently sued for negligence and failure to obtain parental consent before initiating treatment.[1]

Case 2

George, age twenty (at a time when the age of majority was still twenty-one), was playing baseball. He slipped and fell while rounding one of the bases, injuring his ankle. It was painful and rapidly began to swell. George was taken to a local private physician, who determined that the ankle was fractured and required reduction under ether anesthesia. George consented to such treatment and the procedure was carried out without incident. At no time did the physician make any attempt to contact George's parents. The father sued the physician for negligence (for not x-raying the ankle before setting the fracture) and for his failure to first obtain parental consent.[2]

Case 3

Albert, age seventeen, was hitching a ride on a train. On reaching his destination, he attempted to jump off while the train was still in motion. In the process, Albert's coat became entangled in one of the train steps, causing him to be dragged for a considerable distance. He sustained a crushed elbow and a large scalp wound and was taken to the hospital, where the attending physician determined that the wound required immediate surgical attention under general anesthesia. During the procedure, the physician also decided the crushed elbow could not be salvaged, and, with the intention of saving Albert from anesthesia a second time, amputated the arm then and there. At no time had any efforts to contact the parents been made. In addition, Albert had only been advised of the need for attention to his scalp wound and had no prior knowledge of a possible amputation even though he had been conscious up to the time of surgery. Albert's parents sued the surgeon for negligence and failing to first obtain parental consent.[3]

Case 4

Fifteen-year-old Charles was hit by a train, resulting in a severe injury to his left foot. He was taken to a hospital, where he gave the attending physician his name and address. Fifteen minutes thereafter, Charles lost consciousness. After several house physicians examined the foot, they all came to the conclusion that surgical treatment was indicated. An outside surgeon was called in who examined the foot and concurred that an operation was necessary. He was told that the boy's parents were not present nor had they been contacted. The surgeon nonetheless proceeded with the surgery and amputated the foot. A full forty-five minutes had elapsed between Charles's admission to the hospital and the amputation. His parents sued for negligence and failure to first obtain parental consent before initiating treatment.[4]

Did emergencies exist in all of these situations? Were sufficient efforts made to contact the parents before providing treatment? Would any of the physicians be held liable for their failure to obtain prior parental consent?

Definition of an Emergency

While the medical community has often argued over whether a fractured forearm, injured finger, or laceration constitutes an emergency, the courts have been virtually unanimous in their opinions that any such injuries require prompt treatment. In all the preceding cases the physicians were found free of liability for treating the minor without first obtaining parental consent; each situation was adjudged a bona fide emergency. In addition, each physician was also found free of any liability for negligence.

The term "emergency" usually includes not only those situations where the patient is in imminent danger of death but also those situations where a delay in treatment would increase the risk to the patient's health, or treatment is necessary to alleviate physical pain or discomfort. In any emergency, a physician may treat the patient without any consent—either an adult, if he or she is unconscious, or a minor patient in the absence of the parents.

Most states now have statutes specifically addressing emergency care of minors and the issue of parental consent. The vast preponderance of these laws define emergency in extremely broad terms and afford physicians great latitude in exercising their professional judgment as to when an emergency exists and parental consent need not be obtained.

The policy behind these statutes is quite simple: when a minor is in need of urgent medical attention, the physician, or other health service provider, must be *encouraged* to provide treatment free from the fear of liability, thereby enabling the professional to attend to the patient's need without first compromising his or her best judgment. Because of the circumstances surrounding emergency care, and the need for rapid judgments and clinical action, the courts consistently have been and will continue to be extremely reluctant to question professional decisions under these circumstances.

The reader will notice that this section is entitled "Emergency, Urgent, and/or Necessary Health Care." The terminology was selected with a purpose; the health service provider should understand that emergency laws allow treatment for a much broader range of situations than commonly thought. To limit the application of such statutes to strict "emergencies," as that term is commonly defined in medicine, would be unduly restrictive.

While most state emergency statutes are exceptionally broad in definition, the laws in some states, such as Arizona, Idaho, and Montana, are somewhat narrower; reference should always be made to the statute of the reader's locale. Arizona, for example, defines emergency care as procedures necessary for the "treatment of a serious disease, injury, or drug abuse, or to save the life of the patient."[5] These statutes, however, are exceptions. Moreover, courts interpreting even these narrow statutes would acknowledge the need to afford health service providers maximum discretion, and the terms should be interpreted liberally rather than restrictively: as enabling rather than limiting. Unless there is a state statute to the contrary, any health provider may institute treatment without parental consent when the minor patient is in danger of death, or when a delay in treatment pending the contacting of parents and obtaining their consent would increase the risk to the patient's health, broadly defined.

Unlike many other areas of medicine and law, the law defining the scope of emergency health care for minors is clear.

Determining That an Emergency Exists

Before treatment may be given to a minor under emergency circumstances, someone must determine that an "emergency" exists. Not all health service providers are explicitly allowed by statute to make that decision. Only physicians are authorized in some states, while other states include dentists and psychologists as well. Particularly liberal states allow almost any health service professional to make such a determination. Reference should be made to the specific state law in question.

Minors' Consent to Emergency Care

Few states address the issue of whether the minor must consent to the provision of emergency health care. Virginia requires that before rendering emergency treatment to a minor who is fourteen years of age or older and physically capable of giving consent, a health service provider must obtain that minor's consent.[6] Other statutes require the minor's consent by inference. For example, in North Dakota "[a]ny minor may contract for and receive" emergency treatment without parental consent.[7] By definition, minors could not contract for the service unless they were able to give informed consent. (In the statutory table, see also Montana, North Dakota, Rhode Island, Virginia, Wyoming.) The better practice is always to inform the minor of the contemplated procedure, and, if possible, obtain his or her consent for that treatment.

The minor also may be able to consent to the treatment on the basis of his or her status, such as emancipation or level of maturity, thereby offering multiple bases upon which authority to treat in the absence of parents may rest. From a therapeutic standpoint, involving the minor patient in the decision-making process, even when parents are present, especially when the young person is mature enough to give informed consent, is preferred.

It is not clear, however, what would happen if the minor refused treatment. Could the physician treat over the objections of a minor? Would the hospital have to petition a court for permission to treat? Would the physician stand in the place of the parent and therefore have the legal power to override the patient's objections? While no cases on this point were found, it is likely that a court would sustain the ability of a physician to override the objections of the minor, especially if life-saving procedures were contemplated. Such a decision could be based on multiple grounds, including the doctrine of implied parental consent (as discussed earlier), whereby the physician has inherent authority to treat because a rational parent, if present, would consent to the treatment; or the ground that the minor's tender years prevent him or her from making a rational decision, with the refusal itself offering proof of the minor's incompetence; or the ground that in the absence of the parents the physician temporarily takes their place, or stands *in loco parentis*, a term often found in statutes and court decisions. It is best in such situations to seek further legal advice before overriding a mature patient's objection to treatment.

Court Rulings on Health Professionals' Emergency Decisions

Many health service providers believe that professionals' clinical decisions are commonly found to be wanting by the courts, and that they must constantly look over their shoulder in fear that their activities will inevitably become the subject of a malpractice action in a system of law which seems to presume that the patient is always right. Few things could be farther from the truth. Courts rarely question a health professional's decision, especially in emergency situations where clinical decisions must be made quickly.

However, the health professional must exercise sound clinical judgment. He or she must act reasonably and with due regard for the health needs of the minor and the legitimate interests of the parent, especially the parents of a very young minor. For example, in *Zoski* v. *Gaines* nine-year-old Tony was sent to the hospital by his school nurse, who suspected that he had tonsillitis. Tony was examined and told to return to have his tonsils removed. At the appointed time, the boy came back with his fifteen-year-old brother and the procedure was performed. The hospital failed to obtain parental consent. Under such circumstances, the court refused to find an emergency but awarded the parents only six cents in damages, later raised to $600.[8]

In *Moss* v. *Rishworth*, discussed earlier (see "Minors Accompanied by Adults Other than Parents" in chapter 1), Imogene, an eleven-year-old, was taken to a physician by her sister who suspected that Imogene had adenoids. This was confirmed and an operation was performed without first obtaining parental consent. The evidence indicated that, while a prompt operation was indicated, no one, not even the attending physician, contended that any real danger would have resulted had time been taken to consult the parent.[9] Thus, the court refused to dismiss the lawsuit.

Also consider *Dewes* v. *Indian Health Services, etc.*, which did not involve a minor-patient, but is nevertheless useful in analyzing emergency care. Mark, the patient, was involved in a motorcycle accident and fractured both an arm and a leg. He was taken to the hospital but, because of his condition, was not able to give informed consent. However, Mark's parents had been notified by the police and were present at the hospital. Yet the physician failed to take the time to consult with either parent even though, as the court pointed out, the physician had time to take a coffee break. Under such circumstances, where the patient's parents were present in the hospital, and the attending physician had time to drink coffee, the court refused to find emergency circumstances allowing treatment without parental consultation.[10]

Lastly, consider *Tabor* v. *Scobee*, in which the minor patient, Macine, was operated on for appendicitis. During the course of the surgery, the physician discovered that Macine's Fallopian tubes were diseased and summarily removed them without even attempting to first contact her parents. According to the physician, the Fallopian tubes would have had to be removed "within six months anyway if I [the physician] was not mistaken," and he thus sought to have consent implied because of emergency circumstances. The court refused to presume that an emergency existed and left it up to the jury to decide.[11]

It is difficult to formulate absolute rules to assure that the health professional's decision will be ruled beyond reproach. However, based on relevant case law, the following factors should be considered.

First, when the minor is very young and unable to give informed consent, an emergency should be defined somewhat more narrowly. Courts will also prefer that someone, whether patient or parent, provide informed consent whenever possible. As noted above, a nine-year-old with infected tonsils will not be considered an emergency case when the condition will not grow appreciably worse if time is taken to consult the parents.

Second, procedures such as an amputation or the removal of the Fallopian tubes which are irreversible should only be performed in the absence of parental consent when there is no other alternative and attempts to obtain parental consent are not possible or have proven fruitless. Because the results of such procedures are so profound, special care and thought must be taken when they are to be performed without parental consent. However, the reader should be reminded that two of the cases cited at the beginning of this section involved amputations, and in both instances the physicians were found blameless.

Finally, a parent should always be consulted when it is reasonable to do so under the circumstances. This would certainly include parents who are present in the hospital, unless there is urgent need for an immediate life-saving procedure. The parent should be consulted for both the initial treatment and any extensions of treatment, as, for example, when another diseased condition is discovered during the course of an operation; modern anesthetic techniques certainly permit the surgeon to take the time.

Need for a Concurring Opinion

With few exceptions, there is no legal requirement that a physician obtain a concurring medical opinion that an emergency exists before providing treatment to a minor. The "two physician" rule has grown out of the medical profession's practice in emergency situations, not as a result of legislative mandate or judicial opinions.

Only South Carolina, North Carolina, and Oklahoma have second-physician rules, and then only if surgery is contemplated. Even these states waive the requirement when another opinion is not readily available under the circumstances. While the two-physician rule may have a sound clinical basis, there is no legal requirement for it, with the exception of the states listed above.

Efforts at Parental Notification

Individual states differ on what efforts, if any, must be made to contact the parents before emergency treatment may be given to a minor without parental consent. Many states are very permissive, allowing the physician to proceed when *any* attempt at parental contact would result in a delay of treatment resulting in an increased risk to the minor's life or health. In these circumstances, no attempts at notification are required.

Some states, however, do require an initial attempt at parental contact. Arizona requires "reasonably diligent"[12] efforts to be made, while Tennessee requires reasonable efforts if the identity of the parents is readily ascertainable.[13] The reasonableness of an effort to contact a parent will be judged against the exigencies of the circumstances. Is there a great distance between the hospital and the home of the minor? Do the minor's parents have a telephone? How serious is the minor's condition? Does the hospital have a standard protocol, and was that protocol followed?

While most states are silent as to notification after the initiation of treatment, several do have such requirements. Florida, for example, requires that "[n]otification shall be accomplished as soon as possible after the emergency medical care or treatment is administered."[14] In any state, however, the better practice is post-treatment notification if the emergency condition is the only legal basis for the treatment.

Finally, the hospital records should reflect what efforts, if any, were made to contact the parents. If no efforts were made, the reasons should be part of the minor's chart. Florida, for example, requires such documentation.[15]

Emergency Care and Payment Issues

As a general rule, people cannot be required to pay for that to which they did not consent. Theoretically, if the parent did not first consent to the treatment of a minor child, then that parent is not financially responsible. There are, however, strong policy reasons for refuting this logic and requiring the parent's payment for emergency treatment. The reasonable expectation of proper recompense indisputably encourages health care providers to offer emergency health care. There is also a legal argument for this position. Even if a physician provides emergency treatment to a minor without parental consent, under the doctrine of implied consent, had the parents been present they undoubtedly would have consented to the treatment and thus are liable for payment. Indeed, an adult who arrives at a hospital unconscious and receives treatment could not claim lack of consent and avoid payment—consent is implied by the circumstances.

Minors also may have access to various entitlement programs. Medicaid, for example, will pay the medical bills of eligible persons for health services rendered within ninety days of the person's acceptance to the program. So, too, will most private third-party payors when the minor is duly enrolled in a parent's policy. Payment is not contingent upon parents' having given consent; claim forms may be signed well after the treatment.

Emergency Care Summary

Many health service providers believe that a minor must be in imminent and incontrovertible danger of death before emergency care may be given in the absence of parental consent. In fact, such a belief finds no support in law. Judicial opinions addressing cases in which physicians have provided emergency health care to minors consistently endorse the physician's ability to make this determination—a determination nearly beyond reproach. There is, perhaps, no other area of law in which the physician is given such broad latitude.

Minors as Victims of Crimes

Many states have statutes which allow minors who have been the victims of illegal acts to consent to treatment on their own, or at least to receive treatment without parental consent. These statutes usually are applied to those situations where parents cannot be reached quickly and patients could be further harmed by the consequent delay. Examples include a physically abused or sexually molested child, or the minor victim of some other violence. Many of these statutes also explicitly permit X-rays or photographs to be taken in documenting injuries, often at state expense.

The intent of these laws is threefold. The first is to insure prompt treatment of minor victims by allaying health providers' concerns for possible later liability consequent to treating without parental knowledge. But this really is a redundant issue. Not only would a state's emergency care provisions apply to almost any victimized minor who needed care, but also parents have only rarely been awarded damages from a physician solely for treating a child without their permission for any reason and under any circumstances in the absence of negligence (or wrongful treatment). It is our opinion that recovery for care given to a minor harmed as a result of an illegal act, but care to which parents did not consent, is virtually inconceivable. The fact that a particular state might not have a statute on this point should not be seen as disenabling.

As in emergency care, it is also important here to make every reasonable attempt to contact parents before rendering treatment—and to document these efforts in the patient's chart. If parental involvement is not possible or the minor simply refuses to have the parents know, reason dictates that treatment still is to the minor's best benefit and can proceed.

The second purpose of statutes regarding minor victims of crimes is to obtain evidence for possible criminal prosecution. X-rays and other documentation, for example, serve this purpose. Usually this must proceed according to specified protocols, as is the case in each state for victims of rape, child abuse, or child sexual molestation. It is beyond our scope to detail these protocols for every jurisdiction; they are extensive and highly variable. But any emergency room or pediatric clinic should have printed guidelines available if individual clinicians are not familiar with how to proceed themselves. Alternatively, local police or child protective agencies should know these requirements.

The third issue addressed by several of these laws is the question of reimbursement. In order to further encourage prompt treatment and the proper collection of evidence, some statutes require the state to pay for these services. Alternatively, payment may be forthcoming from crime victims' compensation programs in those states having them. In the absence of either of these provisions, providers still may recover from parents or third-party payors according to the same theory as applied to recovery for emergency services: that is, the presumption that reasonable parents would have consented to needed care of their minor child had opportunity permitted, and that their consent was therefore implied.

To help the professional understand consent doctrines for minor crime victims, we particularly recommend the previous section in this chapter on emergency care. Sections in Chapter 2 on emancipated minors and mature minors also may apply. If there is no clear basis on which to treat a minor crime victim without parental consent, further guidance should be sought from a local attorney or hospital counsel.

Sexually Transmitted Diseases

Except for people aged twenty to twenty-five, those who are fifteen to twenty experience the highest incidence of sexually transmitted diseases among all age groups. Nearly every state has a specific statute which allows minors to consent to medical procedures necessary for the detection, diagnosis, and treatment of sexually transmitted diseases without parental consent. The reason is quite simple. Public policy favors the eradication of all communicable diseases, especially those which are of nearly epidemic proportions in the United States, as is the case with gonorrheal and chlamydial infections. In order to effect this policy, most states provide free clinics for the detection and treatment of sexually transmitted diseases, and further require that medical records connected with such treatment be held strictly confidential.

While a minor's legal right to obtain treatment for sexually transmitted diseases without parental consent is not questioned, the reader must be aware that states may differ on such questions as minimum eligible age, post-treatment notification of parents, spouses, or fiancees, and public health reporting requirements.

While most states have no minimum age requirements, a few do mandate parental consent if the minor is less than twelve or fourteen years old. Many do address the question of parental notification after treatment has been given. Some states are quite directive. Illinois, for example, requires the treating professional to make "reasonable efforts" to involve the family. A few other states mandate notification if the minor's life or limb is endangered, or surgical intervention is required. But the vast majority of laws leave the decision about notification to the treating professional's discretion, either simply permitting or specifically encouraging such a step when deemed in the minor's best interests. It should be noted, however, that no state requires notification except in the extraordinary, high-risk circumstances noted above.

The policy of encouraging minors to seek treatment for sexually transmitted diseases would not be served by notification. In allowing minors to consent to treatment without parental consent, state legislatures understood that such a requirement would be likely to dissuade many minors from seeking necessary care. While some legislators may argue that notification of parents after treatment is not the same as requiring their consent before treatment, most minors are not concerned with such abstract notions of personal and informational privacy. They are concerned simply with obtaining treatment for sexually transmitted disease without their parents learning of the fact of the disease—and of the causal behavior. Notification will have no less of a chilling effect than consent on the willingness of minors as a group to seek out treatment.

Finally, any public health reporting requirements applicable to adults regarding the detection of sexually transmitted diseases apply to minors as well. Most states do have such requirements. But these are governed by strict privacy rules which apply to the patient regardless of age. Should public health authorities decide to investigate the case for epidemiological control purposes, the minor can be reassured that the investigating personnel should not violate the rules by knocking on the family's door. The authorities should make every effort to contact the minor in a way which will protect his or her privacy. By and large, public health departments do not investigate the less serious sexually transmitted diseases, including most cases of penicillin-sensitive gonorrhea. There is, however, a reasonable probability that they will investigate cases caused by penicillinase-producing strains of *Neisseria gonorrhoeae* (PPNG). Clinicians should also be aware that most states also require laboratories to report positive syphilis serology tests independent of the patient's or health care provider's knowledge. The question of reported acquired immune deficiency syndrome (AIDS) and positive HTLV III serologies has not yet been resolved, but may introduce a new dilemma as AIDS becomes even more widespread among heterosexual nonintravenous-drug-using populations including sexually active minors.

Contraception

The availability of family planning services to minors is another area in which state statutes have been overridden by federal constitutional law. The Supreme Court has held that contraceptives must be made available to minors and that states may not prohibit such access in the interest of legislating morality.[1]

In this area, most of the states have recognized a minor's right to obtain contraceptives as well as the policy favoring prevention of teen-aged pregnancy and venereal disease through the use of contraceptives and prophylactic devices. Thus many states have adopted statutes mandating that family planning services be provided to all people without regard to sex, age, race, income, number of children, marital status, citizenship, or motive.

Most of the remaining states either have no prohibitory statute or have general medical consent statutes which permit minors to obtain family planning services without parental consent.

Only a few states, such as Florida, have statutes which purport to require parental consent unless the minor is married, a parent, pregnant, or may suffer health hazards if contraceptives are not provided. Such statutes are unconstitutional and may not prevent provision of family planning services to minors not meeting the stated requirements. (See "Abortion" for a more detailed discussion of reproductive privacy rights.)

Finally, Titles XIX (Medical Assistance) and XX (Aid to Families With Dependent Children) of the Social Security Act and Title X of the Family Planning Services and Population Research Act of 1970 require that participating states provide family planning assistance to eligible minors who desire such assistance without regard to marital status, age or parenthood.[2] Parental consent and/or notification is not required or allowed.[3]

The state-by-state table illustrates the nearly uniform acceptance of the constitutional (or, when applicable, federal statutory) mandate that minors be given access to family planning services without parental consent.

Pregnancy Care

Many of the states have specific statutes addressing the ability of a pregnant minor to consent to prevention or treatment of pregnancy. In most such states, a minor "professing to be pregnant" may consent to prevention and treatment, without regard to her age. However, in Delaware, the minor must be at least twelve years old.

Most of the statutes do not define prevention and treatment, although pregnancy testing, pelvic examinations, and prenatal care would certainly be included. However, abortion and sterilization should be regarded as separate issues and are covered in earlier sections of this chapter.

In those states which do not have a statute specifically addressing the pregnant minor, the state's general medical consent statute, as modified by its emancipation and mature-minor doctrines, may permit treatment. Thus, for example, although Louisiana does not have a statute specifically addressing pregnant minors, its liberal consent statute, which essentially permits any minor to consent to any medical treatment, would permit a pregnant minor to consent to treatment of her pregnancy. Even in the absence of a specific statute, however, minors probably have a constitutionally protected privacy right to consent to sex-related health care, and thus there is little doubt that a minor may consent to pregnancy-related health care—assuming, of course, that the minor can give informed consent.

In the context of pregnant minors, the question whether the health care provider should notify the minor's parents arises. While it is usually therapeutically beneficial to involve parents with the minor's consent, such notification is not a prerequisite to treatment, and factors such as possible abuse or expulsion from the home must be considered. The statutes which address this question say that the provider *may (but need not)* notify the minor's parents only when failure to do so would jeopardize the minor's health. (In the state-by-state table, see Kentucky, Maryland, Massachusetts, Minnesota, Missouri, Montana, Oklahoma, Texas.) The Nevada statute requires some efforts to involve the family but does not absolutely require parental consent to, or notification of, pregnancy treatment. Finally, the Missouri and Oklahoma statutes prohibit notification when the minor is found not to be pregnant.

Abortion

The issue of abortion presents complex and difficult problems of constitutional law, many of which are beyond the scope of this book. We present a brief analysis of the major court cases which have settled many of the issues regarding the right of minors to consent to abortions.

The seminal case in this area is *Roe* v. *Wade*, decided in 1973, where the Supreme Court held that women have the constitutionally protected privacy right to determine whether to terminate or continue a pregnancy; a right which may not be unreasonably infringed upon or abridged by the state.[1] The Supreme Court did not rule, however, that a woman has an unfettered constitutional right to an abortion.

Indeed, this point was made clear by the Supreme Court in *Harris* v. *McRae*.[2] In *Harris*, the plaintiffs challenged the constitutionality of the so-called "Hyde Amendment," which cut off federal Medicaid funds for abortions for the medically needy. The plaintiffs contended that if the federal government provided Medicaid funds for childbirth, it was constitutionally required to provide Medicaid funds for abortions; to do otherwise would unfairly weight the choice of poor women toward childbirth. The Supreme Court rejected this contention, holding that while the government could not outlaw abortions, it could, within its discretion, refuse to fund them. In other words, while a poor woman has the privacy right to decide to have an abortion, she does not have the right to an abortion funded by Medicaid, even if the lack of funding would preclude this option. It is worth noting that several states still voluntarily provide public monies for abortions for the medically needy. The courts of several others have ruled that, based on their *state* constitutions, if public funds are provided for childbirth, public funds also must be provided for abortions.[3]

On the whole, subsequent cases regarding abortions have reaffirmed the privacy right enunciated in *Roe*. Thus, the Supreme Court has invalidated statutes which required a husband's consent, or a "cooling off" period before a woman could obtain an abortion, or which required that all abortions after the first trimester be performed in a hospital, or that a physician detail the development of the fetus and the date of possible viability before obtaining a woman's consent to an abortion.[4]

A woman's privacy right to decide whether to have an abortion "is not unqualified," said the Court, "and must be considered against important state interests."[5] The state has two primary interests: the potentiality of human life and the well-being of the woman undergoing an abortion. Thus a state may prohibit abortions once the fetus would be viable outside the mother's womb, except where the life or health of the mother is endangered. A state also may pass reasonable laws that safeguard the health of the patient undergoing an abortion and maintain medical standards. Within the context of *Roe* in 1973, this meant that as a general matter, abortions could be prohibited after the twenty-eighth week of pregnancy but states could not enact statutes which would interfere with a woman's decision to have an abortion within the first trimester—for example, requiring that these abortions take place within a hospital.[6]

In 1983 the Supreme Court again considered several statutes concerning abortions and reaffirmed the trimester analysis, but with slightly different results. To understand completely the decisions, the framework of the *Roe* decision must be expanded upon. In *Roe* the term of a pregnancy was divided into three trimesters, and the state's ability to regulate or forbid abortions depended, in large part, on whether the abortion was to occur within the first, second, or third trimester. Within the first trimester, said the Court, a pregnant woman must be permitted, in consultation with her physician, to decide to have an abortion and to act on that decision free from interference by the state as well as private persons, such as husbands.[7] With the exception of requiring that abortions be performed by licensed physicians, there was little the state could do in terms of regulating first-trimester abortions. This was because the state had no recognizable interest in doing so. First, the fetus was not viable outside the womb, and thus the state had no interest in the potential human life. Second, because "mortality in abortions may be less than mortality in normal childbirth"[8] up to the end of the first trimester, the state had no real interest in safeguarding the health of the mother or in maintaining medical standards by, for example, requiring that all first-trimester abortions take place within a hospital.

Within the second trimester, states were permitted to require that all abortions take place within a hospital setting. Because second-trimester abortion mortality rates were higher than those during the first trimester, such a requirement, said the Court, "reasonably relates [to the state's interest in] the preservation and protection of maternal health."[9] States were not, however, permitted to forbid abortions during the second trimester, because, according to the medical literature, the fetus was not viable outside the womb, and thus the state still had no interest in the potential human life of the fetus. States were permitted to forbid abortions during the third trimester, because the fetus was then viable outside the womb.

The *Roe* trimester analysis was based largely on then-current medical literature, especially medical research regarding viability and mortality rates. The question arose as to what would happen to this analysis in view of medical advances in reducing second-trimester mortality rates and in sustaining the viability of the fetus before the end of the second trimester. The 1983 decisions answered some of these questions.

As an initial matter, the Court reaffirmed its trimester analysis. Thus it is clear that a woman has a nearly unqualified right to opt for an abortion during the first trimester.

The Court's analysis changed somewhat regarding state regulation of abortions during the second trimester. While continuing to hold that the state's interest in health regulation becomes compelling at this point, the Court nevertheless struck down a requirement that all second-trimester abortions occur within a hospital, a requirement that had been held constitutional ten years previously. It did so because medical research indicated that early second trimester abortions could be performed quite safely on an outpatient basis. Thus the regulation was not deemed reasonable. The Court was not presented with the issue of viability outside the womb, at which point states may apparently forbid abortions, although it seems clear that this point is inching earlier because of medical advances.

There may be a contradiction in the Court's reliance on medical science, as pointed out by Justice O'Connor:

> The *Roe* framework . . . is clearly on a collision course with itself. As the medical risks of various abortion procedures decrease, the point at which the State may regulate for reasons of maternal health is moved further forward to actual childbirth. As medical science becomes better able to provide for the separate existence of the fetus, the point of viability is further moved back toward conception.[10]

In view of developing technology, it is possible that the original conceptual framework may need to be revised to protect a woman's right to elect an abortion.

But *Roe* did not address the right of a minor to obtain an abortion without parental consent, and in the wake of this decision, many states passed statutes establishing a parental consent requirement. Proponents argued that mandating parental consent was constitutional, based on the public policy of "safeguarding the authority of the family relationship."[11] In *Planned Parenthood of Missouri* v. *Danforth,* however, the Supreme Court flatly rejected this theory, stating that the policy in favor of parental consent was "no more weighty than the right of privacy of the competent minor mature enough to have become pregnant."[12]

In a series of recent cases, the Supreme Court has established several basic principles and procedural protections regarding a minor's ability to consent to an abortion. First, "a state may not impose a blanket provision . . . requiring the consent of a parent or person *in loco parentis* as a condition for abortion of an unmarried minor."[13]

Second, parental or judicial consent may not be required with respect to *mature* or *emancipated* minors (see chapter 2 for definitions), although it may be required with respect to *immature* minors. Further, state statutes providing for parental or judicial consent must also provide an alternative procedure whereby a pregnant minor may demonstrate that she is sufficiently mature to make the abortion decision herself, or that despite her immaturity, an abortion would be in her best interests.[14] Such procedures must assure anonymity and prompt resolution of the issue. Neither cumbersome procedures nor appeals may be used to restrict "an effective opportunity for an abortion to be obtained."[15] Unless such an alternative procedure is specifically set forth in the statute, the statute is unlikely to withstand constitutional scrutiny. These principles were reaffirmed by the Supreme Court in 1985.

Some states have elected to follow these guidelines, often adopting the following procedures. As a general rule, the consent of one or both parents is required before an abortion may be performed. However, if the adolescent is unwilling to involve her parents, she has the option of applying to the courts and having her case promptly heard by a judge. The judge may only determine whether the minor is or is not sufficiently mature to make an informed decision. If found mature, she may then proceed with the abortion as if she were an adult, and the judge may not veto her decision. Only if she is deemed immature may the judge decide what course is in the minor's best interests. This may range from the ordering of a confidential abortion, at one end of the spectrum, to parental notification of the girl's pregnancy, at the other end.

Most clinical programs providing fertility-related services to teenagers are aware of the precise process for obtaining a hearing and a representing attorney, and provide the minor with detailed counseling accordingly. In some regions, empathetic lawyers have established an "on call" list and provide their services to minors at no or minimal cost. In other regions, the courts appoint counsel for the minor at no cost.

The major issue which has not yet been conclusively resolved by the Supreme Court is whether state statutes may require notification of a minor's parents or guardian before the minor may obtain an abortion. While it is reasonably clear that parental notification requirements, like parental consent requirements, may not be imposed on mature or emancipated minors,[16] it has not yet been definitively resolved whether parental notification statutes must provide the same alternative procedures as specified for consent: namely, that a minor may obtain a prompt judicial determination that she is sufficiently mature to have an abortion without her parents being notified, or that she is immature but notification would not be in her best interests.

In the state-by-state statutory section we have noted when a given statute has already been declared unconstitutional, or when it would not survive such a test and is clearly unconstitutional even though no such declaration has yet been made for the specific statute in question. In these latter cases, it may be appropriate for the provider to seek specific legal advice and possibly to seek a judicial ruling on the validity of a state statute which may unconstitutionally limit minors' access to abortions. In addition, the Supreme Court is likely to issue additional rulings in the future which may alter the rules discussed above. Those providers who are involved in counseling adolescents about such matters should keep alert.

Proxy Consent for an Abortion

Under no circumstances may a parent legally compel a competent minor offspring to undergo an abortion against the minor's wishes.[17] A markedly different question arises when the minor is incompetent to consent to an abortion due to mental retardation, or severe emotional disturbance. Under these circumstances, the substitution of parental consent is probably appropriate, and the need for a court order limited.

When the mental incapacity of the minor is beyond question, there is generally no role for a court to play, and the consent of the parent is sufficient. One court, in rejecting the notion that a judicial hearing should be required in all cases, stated: "[A] judge should [not even be given the opportunity to] invoke his or her own moral, philosophical, theological and sociological precepts in deciding whether [abortion] should take place."[18] Although this case involved a twenty-five-year-old woman with the mental age of a two-year-old, there is no reason to believe that the judge would have reached a different conclusion had the young woman been a minor. Indeed, the state's *parens patriae* role as the final protector of the incompetent is the same, whether at twenty-six, sixteen, or even six years of age.

If, however, there is any question regarding the minor's competency, a judicial hearing should be convened. If the minor is, in fact, adjudged to be incompetent, it is most likely that the court will allow the parents to decide. On the other hand, if the minor is ruled competent, only she and her physician may make the decision to have or not to have an abortion; no third party may intervene.

Last, if a minor is incompetent and no parent or legal guardian is available to consent to an abortion (as might occur with an institutionalized adolescent), a court order should be obtained which both confirms the incompetency of the minor and specifically permits the abortion to go forward. Under these circumstances, the state, under the doctrine of *parens patriae*, takes over the guardian role in deciding what course is in the minor's best interest.

This issue, however, is not settled. The health care provider, when confronted with parents who seek to substitute their consent for their minor child's on the basis of the child's incompetency, should seek legal advice on relevant state law.

Sterilization

Sterilization presents a very different situation because of its irrevocability and because minors, no matter how mature, may indeed be incapable of adequately evaluating such a procedure and deciding whether or not to have it performed. Moreover, there is a potential for the exertion of undue influence over minors (and adult women), who may be convinced to consent to sterilization in conjunction with delivery of their children.

To protect against this problem, federal regulations provide that federal reimbursement is not available under any circumstances for sterilization procedures performed on a person unless he or she is at least twenty-one, is mentally competent, and has given informed consent at least 30 days but not more than 180 days before the operation.[1]

Many of the states have statutes which specifically address sterilization and impose a minimum age of eighteen for the operation to be performed. In cases involving sterilization, because of the seriousness and irrevocability of the procedure and the potential for undue influence in the decision-making process, the federal and state rules should be followed to the letter. In states without specific statutes, minors should not be permitted to consent for sterilization. We note, however, in the only case we found where a physician was sued for sterilizing a minor on the minor's own consent, that the court found the physician blameless because the minor was sufficiently mature to give informed consent.[2]

Sterilization of the Retarded—A Special Problem

Above we discussed whether a minor may voluntarily seek out and obtain a sterilization. Here we consider whether mentally incompetent postpubescent minors may be sterilized. The typical case would be the following:

> Mr. and Mrs. Jones have a fifteen-year-old daughter, Sonya, whose mental development is seriously retarded: she has the competence of a three-year-old. Sonya's physical development, however, is age-appropriate and she has become a young woman. Sonya experiences considerable discomfort during her menstrual cycle. She does not seem to understand the source of her pain and often appears confused and disoriented during this time. She is unable to understand the need for personal hygiene and often removes her feminine napkins. In addition, she refuses to attend school during her cycle, preferring to simply lie in bed. Mr. and Mrs. Jones seek to relieve Sonya of her discomfort. They are also quite concerned that her lack of mental development and understanding of the reproductive process may lead her to become pregnant.

The issues raised by Sonya's situation are extremely complex and raise a host of deep, divisive moral and ethical debates about the rights of incompetents. The issues raised by the sterilization of incompetents must be viewed against a historical backdrop. As the court stated in *In re Grady*:

> Sterilization has a sordid past in this country—especially from the viewpoint of the mentally retarded. In the early part of this century many states enacted compulsory sterilization laws as an easy answer to the problems and costs of caring for the misfortunate of society. Lawmakers may have sincerely believed that the social welfare would improve if fewer handicapped people were born, but they were too quick to accept unproven scientific theories of eugenics. In the United States Supreme Court, a compulsory sterilization law withstood a challenge that such legislation unconstitutionally infringes upon liberty protected by the due process clause. In *Buck* v. *Bell*, 274 U.S. 200, 47 S. Ct. 584, 71 L. Ed. 1000 (1927), the Court upheld a law authorizing the compulsory sterilization of a mentally impaired woman for no more compelling reason than to prevent another generation of "imbeciles."[3]

It was not until 1942, when the Supreme Court of the United States declared unconstitutional the Oklahoma law which permitted the forced sterilization of "habitual criminals," that the Court recognized procreation as a fundamental right and thus, in effect, outlawed the involuntary sterilization of any individual. Courts approach this irreversible operation involving the basic human right to procreate[4] with extreme caution. Indeed, this caution has led a number of courts to determine that in the absence of express legislative authorization, no court may order the sterilization of an incompetent minor.[5] This view, however, seems to be on the wane,[6] and it has been criticized as an "abdication of the judicial function"[7] because, under the doctrine of *parens patriae*, courts have always had the inherent power to protect those who cannot protect themselves due to incompetency. We can expect to see more courts willing to entertain applications for the sterilization of incompetent minors.

Recently, courts have ruled that the sterilization of an incompetent minor may be in the minor's best interest. The courts, however, clearly not wanting to regress to the time when the sterilization of the incompetent could be effected for reasons of simple expediency, have set up rigorous criteria which must be met before such an application would be granted. The standards set forth below are taken from a number of cases from different states. The reader must check the locale in which he or she practices to determine if cases will be heard by the court, and, if so, the reasons for which a court would grant such a request.

Factors a Court Probably Would Consider

1. The sterilization must be shown by clear and convincing evidence to be in the best interests of the incompetent.
2. The incompetent must be afforded a full judicial hearing to consider the application, and a guardian must be appointed to represent his or her interests.
3. A comprehensive medical, psychological, and social evaluation must be presented to the court.
4. The individual must be shown to be incompetent and unable to understand reproduction and contraception, and it must be shown that this condition is, in all likelihood, permanent.
5. The incompetent must be shown capable of reproduction and unable to care for her offspring. According to one court, it does not have to be shown that pregnancy is likely.
6. Sterilization must be the only means of contraception. In this regard, it must be shown why other less drastic forms of contraception would not be appropriate.
7. On balance, it must be shown that the incompetent will suffer more physical and psychological harm from a pregnancy and birth than from sterilization.
8. The advisability of sterilization at the time of the application rather than at some future date must be documented.
9. The person seeking the sterilization must demonstrate that the application is in good faith without concern for public finances or convenience.
10. It must be demonstrated that a less drastic form of contraception will not be shortly available.
11. The court must be satisfied that science is not poised at the threshold of a discovery which may render the incompetent more able to participate in this decision.

12. Finally, one court required that the procedures be medically necessary or medically essential.[8]

The law is extremely unstable and is subject to sudden change. For example, science, in the very near short term, may develop a safe form of contraception (not requiring daily use for effectiveness) which may solve the practical problems of assuring that incompetents are protected against unwanted pregnancies without requiring them to be surgically sterilized. Should that happen, it is unlikely that any court would permit the sterilization of an incompetent person. The health care provider, faced with the sterilization of an incompetent, must first seek the assistance of counsel.

Substance Abuse

Most states specifically allow minors to obtain medical procedures and psychological services necessary for the detection, diagnosis, and treatment of substance abuse on their own consent and without that of parents. This reflects clear public policy interests in controlling and eradicating this serious and ubiquitous problem. States recognize that adolescent minors are particularly at risk and are unlikely to seek out help if not offered confidential care.[1]

While the majority of state statutes address both alcohol abuse and drug abuse in a similar fashion, this is not universal. Some statutes speak only to drug abuse or only to alcoholism.[2] In referring to the statutory tables, readers should take particular note of this fact. But we are of the opinion that even when statutes do not speak to alcoholism, provisions for "drug" abuse could be interpreted to include alcohol as well. Alcohol use to the point of habituation or addiction by an adolescent would more than likely qualify as "drug" abuse.

Another point which should be noted is that some states have a minimum age below which parental consent is required. Usually this is in the range of twelve to fourteen years. When such is the case, it, too, is noted in the state-by-state rundown.[3]

Ten states do not have any statutes addressing substance abuse at all. But even here, as well as in states having only partial laws, there is little risk in treating minors without parental consent for either a drug or alcohol abuse problem. Often there is some other basis for treatment. The minor may be emancipated or mature, or the health need may rise to the level of an emergency. Laws governing unemancipated minors living away from home (e.g., runaways) may also apply. Moreover, as we have noted on several other occasions, there have been no court decisions in the last twenty years in which a physician has been found liable for treating a minor over age fifteen on his or her consent alone for any purpose, as long as the treatment was both for the benefit of the minor and deemed necessary according to accepted standards of medical practice. Certainly, the treatment of substance abuse would meet these criteria.

Further, at least one legal scholar has stated that even in the absence of permissory laws, adolescents in need of substance abuse services, but who refuse parental involvement, nonetheless may consent, since "the societal and personal consequences as to the child of the addiction are so profound." The need to curb substance abuse among the young clearly outweighs any benefits which may be realized by parental consent requirements.[4]

Solving the question of consent does not necessarily solve the question of notification. States vary considerably on parental notification once treatment is sought by or provided to a minor. Some definitively prohibit disclosure,[5] while others leave this to the treating professional's discretion.[6] Yet others require notification if the minor either is still in treatment after a specified period of time, usually three months, or is hospitalized.[7] And a last group permits parental notification about definitively afflicted minors, but prohibits it if suspected substance abuse is ruled out.[8]

In programs where there are no applicable notification rules because the state statute is silent, sound policy dictates against notification without the minor's concurrence except in extraordinary circumstances (as could be the case when an adolescent experiences a serious overdose reaction with risk to life). Young people in need of substance abuse treatment will be most reluctant to seek it if parents must know.

From the medical management perspective, however, one cannot successfully treat an abusing adolescent who is still living at home without family involvement; they are all implicated in the problem. It is also true that many of these youngsters do want their parents' active support but do not know how to go about telling them out of fear of rejection or punitive retribution. While confidential access to a treatment facility is essential to attract a young person who needs care, once the health provider has gained the patient's trust, usually within two or three visits, it commonly becomes possible to negotiate how and when parents will be told. It also is worth noting parenthetically that parents commonly are already aware of the problem, but do not, themselves, know how to broach the subject; all the members of the family enter into a conspiracy of silence. From a therapeutic vantage point, then, the legal parameters governing parental notification within a particular state often are not at issue.

Drug and Alcohol Records—Special Privacy Regulations

Any youth-serving program or agency which provides drug or alcohol counseling or treatment and receives any sort of federal funding is subject to very strict regulations regarding the release and dissemination of the minor's records. Failure to abide by these regulations could subject a program to a fine or possible civil lawsuit. Thus the regulations are addressed at length below.

To enhance the attractiveness and effectiveness of drug and alcohol abuse treatment programs, Congress enacted 21 U.S.C. §1175, which mandates that patients' records in drug and alcohol programs (substance abuse programs) receiving any type of federal aid are to be strictly confidential. The Department of Health and Human Services has enacted 42 C.F.R. Part 2, regulations which define a program's obligations under §1175. Information concerning the "identity, diagnosis, prognosis or treatment" of any patient may only be disclosed in specific, limited situations. Violation of any of the provisions concerning confidentiality is a criminal offense, punishable by a fine of up to $5,000.[1]

Initially, three points must be clear to understand the extent of §1175 and its regulations. The term "patient" refers to any individual who has ever applied for, been referred to, or been diagnosed and treated by the substance abuse program.[2] Thus an individual who is no longer in the program or who only applied for admittance is considered a patient for the purposes of these regulations and is to be accorded the required confidentiality.

The term "patient information" includes all knowledge any staff member may have about a patient. The information need not be recorded. It may not have been received from the patient directly. Any knowledge of a patient acquired in connection with a drug or alcohol abuse treatment system is to be accorded confidential status.[3] The prohibition against disclosure includes information on the physical whereabouts of a patient, his or her attendance at the program, or an individual's status as a patient. Implicit or negative disclosures are equally prevented. The identity of the seeker is of no consequence, as is the fact that the seeker may already have the information sought.[4]

The regulations may apply to records, even when they are unrelated to drug abuse counseling, and even when the patient initially comes to a program for reasons unrelated to substance abuse but is diagnosed as having a substance abuse problem. In *Commissioner of Social Services* v. *David R. S.*,[5] a putative father, who was being sued for paternity, sought the medical records of the mother pertaining to examinations, consultations, birth control, and other matters from The Door, a youth center which provided a variety of services including substance abuse counseling. The Door resisted disclosure, arguing that the records were protected by the federal regulations. The father argued that because the mother had initially gone to the program for sex-related health care, not substance abuse treatment, the regulations did not apply, and, even if they did apply, only those records pertaining to substance abuse treatment were protected. The New York Court of Appeals rejected the father's arguments. It stated:

> Patient records maintained by a drug abuse treatment center which is assisted by an agency of the United States are not be be denied the shelter of statutory confidentiality where the center made a diagnosis for drug abuse, notwithstanding that the patient first sought non-drug-related services from the center and that the records sought to be disclosed pertain to other than a drug-related condition.[6]

Finally, the standards presented by the regulations are the minimum requirements which must be met. Any ethical standards of a profession which go beyond the Department of Health and Human Services (HHS) regulations are still to be met by the individuals involved.

Disclosure with Patient's Consent

Information concerning a patient's involvement in a drug and/or alcohol abuse treatment program may be given to particular people and agencies with the patient's consent. If the minor patient has the legal capacity under state law to obtain the services of the treatment program, any consent required for disclosure under the federal regulations may *only* be given by the minor and not the parent.[7] If state law requires parental consent for treatment, the minor applying for treatment must consent to the notification of his or her parents before the parents are contacted by the treatment program.

Consent is required before information may be given to a patient's family, attorney, third-party payors and funding sources, or medical personnel.[8] Treatment may not be made contingent on consent to information disclosure. To be valid, consent must be voluntarily given.

Consent to disclosure must be written. It must contain the names of the treatment program, the person or agency receiving the information, and the patient involved. The purpose or need for disclosure and the extent of information to be disclosed must be clearly stated. A statement that consent may be revoked at any time and a specification of the date, event, or condition on which consent will expire without express revocation must be made. The signature of the patient (and parent if required) and the date must appear.[9] No disclosure may be made if any item is missing from the consent form.

Any disclosure which is made by a program must conform to the patient's consent, and must be accompanied by a statement informing the recipient of the confidential nature of the information, and notifying the recipient that any further disclosure of the information is illegal.

If consent has been given for disclosure to a person or agency not specifically provided for by the HHS regulations as outlined above, the program director may permit disclosure if (1) there is no question of the validity and voluntary grant of consent; (2) granting the request will not damage the relationship between the program and the individual patient, or the general functioning of the program; and (3) granting the information request will not be harmful to the patient. Disclosures to public assistance agencies have been specifically deemed beneficial to the patient.[10]

Disclosure Without Consent

Situations meriting disclosure of information without the patient's consent are specifically described and very limited. Disclosure of information to medical personnel when necessary to meet a "bona fide medical emergency" is permitted. Information, other than patient identity data, may also be disclosed for the purpose of scientific research, management or financial audits, and program evaluations.[11] Any other disclosure without the patient's consent must be carefully and individually evaluated.

Child abuse. Without question "[t]he relationship between the federal confidentiality rules and state laws mandating the reporting of child abuse and neglect [is] a source of great controversy and confusion"[12] because they often conflict with each other; the federal regulations prohibit disclosure and state law mandates it when the substance abuse patient is abusing a child. Simply put, the federal confidentiality regulations supersede state reporting requirements regarding child abuse. Making a report of child abuse may be prohibited unless certain conditions are met.

Reporting is permissible under any of the following circumstances:

1. A court order permitting disclosure is obtained (procedure described below).
2. A report can be made without identifying the patient as recipient of alcohol or drug treatment (this could include an anonymous report or a report from a program which is not, by definition, a substance abuse program, for example, the emergency room of a hospital).
3. When the patient is the victim of the abuse, the consent of the patient is obtained.
4. A report is made to a child-protective agency with which the program has entered into a qualified service organization contract.[13]

When a physician determines that he or she cannot report a case of child abuse because of the federal regulations, we strongly urge that legal counsel be consulted and a court-ordered disclosure, as described below, sought. Failure to do so could result in the physician being held civilly liable should the child suffer further as a result.

Court-ordered disclosure. In particular and very narrow circumstances, a court may order the disclosure of information which is ordinarily confidential. Even within these circumstances, the information which can be disclosed is limited. Only records kept by the treatment program itself may be ordered disclosed. Thus records kept by auditors, or in connection with research, cannot be affected by court-ordered disclosure.[14] Furthermore, unless the patient involved has offered testimony about the content of his or her treatment by the program, only objective data, such as facts and dates of enrollment, can be ordered disclosed. Finally, only the data necessary to fulfill the purpose for which the order is issued can be disclosed.

Any person with a legally recognized interest in obtaining disclosure may apply for a court order.

The application should be instituted under a fictitious name and not the name of the patient. Both the patient and the program involved must be accorded "appropriate notice and an opportunity to appear in person or to file a response," even if they are not parties to the action involved.

Unless the patient requests an open hearing, or the court determines such a hearing is consistent with the "public interest and the proper administration of justice," all hearings will be held in judge's chambers.

An order to disclose information will only be issued if "good cause" is found. Good cause will be assessed by weighing the public interest and the need for disclosure against the injury to the patient, the physician-patient relationship, and the treatment program.

The existence of other competent sources of information or evidence should result in a denial of the application. Similarly, evidence that disclosure will adversely affect the successful treatment of the involved patient, or of other patients, or will impair the effectiveness of the program or other programs similarly situated, should result in the denial of the court order.

An order requiring disclosure must be designed to keep disclosure to a minimum. Only the parts of the patient's record deemed essential to fulfill the purpose of the order can be disclosed, and the person whose need for information is the basis of the order is the only one to whom disclosure will be made.[15]

Release of information to law enforcement agencies. Any disclosure of information sought by law enforcement personnel to investigate or prosecute any patient must be authorized by a court order. A mere request or a subpoena of information must be refused if unaccompanied by a court order issued in accordance with the HHS rules. If there is a court order, the information may be disclosed, but only to the extent of complying with the purpose of which the court order was granted.

Applications for court-order disclosure made by any investigative, law enforcement, or prosecutorial agency are handled slightly differently than those described above.

Unless the program itself is being investigated, it must be notified of the application and afforded an opportunity to appear and be heard. Any application should be denied unless the court specifically finds that the program has been afforded the opportunity to be represented by independent counsel.

The application for disclosure may only be granted if the court finds that: (1) the crime involved was extremely serious, threatening loss of life or great bodily harm; (2) there is a reasonable likelihood that the records will disclose material information or evidence of substantial value in connection with the investigation or prosecution; (3) there is no other practical way of obtaining the information or evidence; and (4) the injury to the physician–patient relationships in the program and other programs similarly situated, and the harm done to these programs' ability to attract and retain patients, is outweighed by the public interest in disclosure.[16]

Any order granted to investigative, law enforcement, or prosecutorial agencies should be limited to the information specifically needed. No order may be issued requiring a program to release a patient's records in general.

If the program itself is being investigated, whether by an administrative, regulatory, supervisory, investigative, law enforcement, or prosecutorial agency, the application may be granted without notice to the program. The program, however, must have an opportunity to seek revocation or amendment of the order.

Any disclosure during the investigation of a program must protect patient identities to the maximum extent possible. Names or other identifying information must be expunged from any documents which become part of the public record.[17]

Conclusion

In view of the gradations of the regulations concerning confidentiality, and the seriousness of the penalties for improper disclosure, any requests for information or questions about disclosure should be referred to an attorney.

Mental Health Care

The question of when minors may consent to mental health treatment is necessarily related to when a parent may consent to voluntary treatment on behalf of a minor child. In turn this issue must be subdivided into hospitalized patients and those being treated on an outpatient basis. Most states have statutes regarding hospitalization; few address ambulatory care.

Our discussion here, however, does *not* include minors seeking treatment for substance abuse problems. Most states have statutes specifically addressed to that point, which have been dealt with in the previous section.

Voluntary Hospitalization

The placement of minors in mental hospitals raises two separate questions. The first relates to the authority of parents or other adults to voluntarily commit minors. The second asks whether minors have any authority to commit themselves or to terminate their commitment if it was initiated by another.

While the United States Supreme Court has upheld the right of parents (or legal guardians) to seek placement of their minor child in a mental hospital, this is not without qualification. Minors also have certain rather minimal constitutional protections of their own relating to process and procedure.[1] These are to ensure that hospitalization is both necessary and for the minor's benefit; not simply the result of parental interests in sequestering a troublesome adolescent.

Accordingly, when a parent applies for admission on behalf of a minor child, a psychiatrist empowered to refuse admission if not indicated must independently evaluate the minor's mental and emotional condition and treatment needs. This evaluation must include an interview with the minor alone and a careful probe of his or her background using all available sources of information including parents, schools, and social agencies. In addition, the minor's continuing need for commitment must be periodically reviewed by a similarly independent procedure, although the Supreme Court has not specified the frequency with which this must be carried out.[2]

These requirements are the minimum necessary to meet constitutional standards. Individual states are free to impose additional protections by statute or regulation. A number have taken such steps. For example, New Mexico, South Dakota, Texas, and Wisconsin require that minors be informed of their right to object to commitment and to have a hearing. Other states have specified the frequency with which the need for continuing hospitalization must be reviewed. In Arizona this must be every ten days; in Montana voluntary admission is automatically terminated after one year and a case review is necessary for readmission.

A few states have additional rules for minors who are wards of the state. The question of what persons other than parents (or legal guardians) are authorized to seek voluntary commitment of a minor will not be detailed in the state-by-state table, but answers should be well known to mental hospital administrators.

Most states also permit minors beyond a certain age to commit themselves voluntarily. For example, a youth need only be age twelve in Georgia or fourteen in Alabama to consent to his or her own admission, but in Florida the minimum age is seventeen years. Other states require a combination of parental consent—or notice—and the minor's consent if he or she has reached a certain age. Another alternative permits application by either a parent *or* an eligible minor. These qualifications are detailed for those states in which they apply in the state-by-state table.

General provisions governing emancipated and mature minors and the age of majority for health care consent also apply to mental health. Some states specifically take statutory note, as in Idaho for emancipated minors and Mississippi (among others) for married minors regardless of age.

A number of states protect minors by mandating judicial review in all cases of commitment regardless of who initiated the application process. Florida, for example, requires either that parents institute *involuntary* commitment proceedings or that there be a court hearing to verify that the minor's consent was indeed voluntary. (Involuntary commitment also requires a specific legal process to insure that the patient's interests are independently represented and protected, whether he or she is minor or adult.) Hawaii permits admission of minors fifteen to seventeen years old only after involuntary commitment proceedings unless the minor signs the application before a family court officer.

In most states, minors may terminate their voluntary commitment at any time (even if they were initially admitted by a parent), as long as they have reached the state's age of consent for admission in the first place, as previously discussed. Several states also permit minors under the age of consent to object to continuation of commitment and receive a hearing. There may be the companion requirement that the initial applicant, if other than the patient himself or herself, must be notified of the minor's intent to terminate care.

The rules governing a minor's admission to a mental hospital are variable and complex. The laws in each state will need to be looked to for direction.

Outpatient Treatment

A minority of states have enacted statutes specifically addressing the ability of minors to consent to outpatient mental health treatment. In the absence of a specific statute, a state's rules governing medical consent in general, including emancipated and mature minors, would most likely apply by analogy to outpatient mental health services. Thus the psychologist or social worker could provide services—even independently of a physician.

It would be anomalous indeed if the law permitted a minor to consent to a surgical procedure, or to commitment to a mental health facility, but denied the same minor the capacity to consent to outpatient mental health counseling. Moreover, it is hard to imagine any policy reasons denying a minor the right to consent to counseling. Indeed, as we have seen, the legislatures and courts have repeatedly waived the requirement of parental consent in sensitive health areas such as drug or alcohol abuse, treatment for sexually transmitted diseases, and other sex-related health care. Little could be more sensitive than the revelations of one's innermost thoughts to a therapist. As the court stated in *Ceasar* v. *Mountanos*:

> Psychotherapy probes the core of the patient's personality. The patient's most intimate thoughts and emotions are exposed during the course of the treatment. "The psychiatric patient confides [in his

> therapist] more utterly than anyone else in the world. . . . [H]e lays bare his entire self, his dreams, his fantasies, his sin, and his shame." . . . The patient's innermost thoughts may be so frightening, embarrassing, shameful or morbid that the patient in therapy will struggle to remain sick, rather than to reveal those thoughts even to himself. The possibility that the psychotherapist could be compelled to reveal those communications to anyone . . . can deter persons from seeking needed treatment and destroy treatment in progress.[3]

Thus it is likely that a court would view the benefit of confidentiality to a minor in need of mental health care as of a higher order than the benefit of requiring parental consent. This would probably extend to notification of the parent that the minor is in therapy. Further support to the right of a minor to consent to health care can be gleaned from the fact that nearly every state allows a minor to consent to substance abuse services. It would seem almost absurd to hold that the same minor, cured of the drug affliction, could not continue to consent to mental health treatment for other emotional problems. Finally, the constitutional right to privacy may also apply to communications between a patient and therapist, lending additional support to the right of a minor to consent to outpatient mental health treatment.[4]

Refusal of Treatment

When a minor refuses admission for in-patient mental health care, many states nonetheless allow the minor to be committed, as long as parental consent is obtained. Even in those states where the parents cannot "voluntarily" commit a minor on their consent alone, other procedures exist for involuntary commitment. States generally permit involuntary commitment of both minors and adults if the need for emergency psychiatric hospitalization is evident and attested to by one or two physicians. Customarily, a court hearing must be convened very shortly after an involuntary commitment, and the patient may be retained only upon a court order.

A separate question, however, is raised when a minor is involuntarily hospitalized but refuses or resists the administration of drugs or other therapies. The Supreme Court has recognized that commitment to a mental facility deprives the minor of substantial liberty, and the Court has stipulated that commitment can only occur after certain due process protections are satisfied. (Many critics argue that these are woefully inadequate.)

Similarly, the administration of electroshock therapy, and, to a lesser extent, powerful psychothropic and sedative drugs, can also deprive the patient of some liberty interest, albeit not as a substantial an interest as does involuntary commitment. The hospitalized patient who resists treatments must be afforded some protections, but how much is the subject of considerable debate, and varies from state to state, even for adults.[5] But a few comments can be made. First, unless there is an emergency or the finding of incapacity to understand treatment, a mental patient, minor or adult, may refuse the administration of drugs or electroshock. Second, once the patient refuses, adequate professional review of the mode of treatment must occur, although it is unlikely that the patient would be entitled to a court hearing (unless such a hearing was specifically required under state law). But even with such a review, it is unlikely that a minor's objection to treatment, particularly if the minor were very young, would be afforded the same legal weight as would the refusal of an adult. The patient's mental status would also have a bearing; the psychotic patient has less persuasive power than the one who is reasonably well grounded in reality.

Many psychothropic agents commonly have dysphoric side effects, and adolescents on such medication frequently object to the treatment. However, in light of the improved clinical outcome that can occur with these drugs, and in light of the absence of definitive law on the issue, the decisions of the treating psychiatrist, competently made, as to what medication regimen is in the minor patient's best interests will usually prevail. Unfortunately, there is a tendency to sometimes utilize these drugs as a type of pharmacologic straightjacket in managing the acting-out adolescent. But this dilemma is better addressed through the development and maintenance of high clinical standards than through the law.

CHAPTER 4

Special Situations

Minors as Research Subjects

Considerable debate surrounds the use of human subjects for research. The profound ethical, philosophical, and moral dilemmas related to the issue have led to widely diverging schools of opinion and blurred legal questions. But in 1983, following extensive study and the development of a set of recommendations by the National Commission for the Protection of Human Subjects of Biomedical and Behavioral Research, the Department of Health and Human Services issued specific regulations governing federally funded research in which adults and children serve as research subjects.[1] These regulations have answered many of the previous questions regarding the legal propriety of utilizing minors as research subjects.

Applicability

The HHS regulations apply "to all research involving human subjects conducted by [a federal] grant, contract, cooperative agreement or fellowship."[2] Consequently, these regulations do not apply to *all* research, but, because of the broad extent to which research is supported by governmental funds, and because of the practical need to have uniform protocols, they are currently viewed as the standard.

Research activities are defined in the regulations simply as "a systematic investigation, designed to develop or contribute to generalizable knowledge."[3] The Commission defined research somewhat more completely as "an activity designed to test an hypothesis, permit conclusions to be drawn, and thereby . . . develop or contribute to generalizable knowledge."[4]

The Commission also provided a framework for distinguishing research from medical practice. It stated that the latter "refers to interventions that are designed *solely* to enhance the well-being of an individual patient or client and that have a reasonable expectation of success" [emphasis added].[5] The Commission went on to state that "[t]he fact that a procedure is experimental, in the sense of new, untested or different, does not automatically place it in the category of research," although "a major innovation [should] be incorporated into a formal research project."[6]

The HHS regulations go one step further in setting forth a list of activities which are defined as "exempt" research and to which the regulations do not apply. These include, for example, certain types of educational testing and research; research involving survey or interviewing procedures in which the subjects remain anonymous and would not be harmed if their responses became known; research that does not deal with sensitive aspects of behavior; research involving the observation of public behavior; and research involving the collection of existing data.[7] These exemptions are generally applicable to research involving children as well. Research involving survey or interviewing procedures, however, must be reviewed and approved by an institutional review board (IRB).

The IRB is at the heart of the HHS regulations. Each institution engaged in research covered by the regulations must have an IRB composed of at least five members whose task it is to assure that the research projects conducted under the auspices of that institution are done in conformity with the regulations. It is not our intent to set forth the functions of the IRB in detail. Readers engaged in research are certainly well aware of its operation. Suffice it to say here that its principal function is to pass on research protocols and to assure that human subjects are adequately protected in relation to the risk-benefit ratio, selection as subjects, and in giving informed consent to serve as a research subject.[8] It is the last function which is the core of our concern.

Informed Consent Generally

The regulations describe, in detail, the information which must be given to persons who are to serve as research subjects before obtaining their informed consent. This must be in writing and include the following:

- A description of the research and its purposes.
- Any foreseeable risks or discomforts to the subject.
- Any benefits that the subject or others may realize.
- Appropriate alternative treatments, if any.
- The extent to which confidentiality will be maintained.
- If the research involves more than minimal risk, a statement as to whether compensation is being paid, and what medical procedures are provided if injury occurs.
- The name of a person whom the subject may contact for more information and to whom subjects should report possible research-related injuries.
- A statement that participation is voluntary and that refusal to participate will not result in any sanctions.
- A statement that the subject may discontinue participation at any time without prejudice.

An IRB, however, may waive or modify these informed-consent requirements when: (1) the research involves no more than minimal risk to the subject (that is, the risk of harm is no greater than those risks encountered in daily life or during the performance of routine physical or psychological tests); *and* (2) the subject's rights or welfare will not be adversely affected; *and* (3) as a practical matter, the research cannot be conducted without waiver or modification.[9]

Parental Consent Requirements

As a general matter, minors may not serve as research subjects without parental permission and, in most cases, their own "assent." If the proposed procedure involves more than minimal risk to the minor without the prospect of him or her receiving direct therapeutic benefit, the consent of *both* parents must be obtained where reasonably possible, unless one parent is unknown, incompetent, or not available, or only one parent has the legal responsibility for the care and custody of the child.[10] If the research presents only a minimal risk and/or holds out the promise of direct therapeutic benefit, the IRB may deem the permission of one parent sufficient.

There are situations, however, in which the IRB is permitted to waive entirely, or in part, the requirement of parental permission, or where parental permission is not required. These exceptions are of particular relevance for research with adolescents. If the requirement for parental permission is "not a reasonable requirement," then permission may be waived, but an alternative procedure must be substituted to protect the minor.[11] Research in child abuse is given as an example of when the requirement would not be reasonable. Although additional examples were provided by the Commission upon which HHS relied so heavily, the examples were not included in the final regulations.

The regulations do not define the alternative procedures which must be substituted to protect minors when parental permission is waived. They state that the substitute mechanism "would depend upon the nature and purpose of the [research], the risk and anticipated benefit to the [minors], and their age, maturity, status, and condition.[12] Some additional guidance may be gleaned from the following commentary in the Commission report:

> There is no single mechanism that can be substituted for parental permission in every instance. In some cases the consent of mature minors should be sufficient. In other cases court approval may be required. The mechanism invoked will vary with the research and the age, status and condition of the prospective subjects.
>
> [A]ssent of . . . mature minors should be considered sufficient with respect to research about conditions for which they have legal authority to consent on their own to treatment.
>
> An appropriate mechanism for protecting such subjects might be to require that a clinic nurse or physician, unrelated to the research, ex-

> plain the nature and the purpose of the research . . . emphasizing that participation is unrelated to provision of care.
>
> Another alternative might be to appoint a social worker, pediatric nurse, or physician to act as surrogate parent when the research is designed, for example, to study neglected or battered children. Such surrogate parents would be expected to participate not only in the process of soliciting the children's cooperation but also in the conduct of the research, in order to provide reassurance for the subject and to intervene or support their desires to withdraw if participation becomes too stressful.[13]

There is no requirement for parental permission (nor the need to request a waiver) when the minor "ha[s] attained the legal age for consent to treatment or procedures involved in the research, under the applicable law of the jurisdiction in which the research will be conducted."[14] Minors with sexually transmitted diseases, for example, can consent to research procedures relating to such conditions because they may consent to treatment for sexually transmitted diseases, usually without regard to age. The same reasoning applies to research on substance abuse, pregnancy, or contraception.

Whether a minor may consent to participate in research which is not directly related to his or her treatment remains somewhat ambiguous. This could include, for example, a questionnaire to be completed by a minor who has undergone an abortion.[15] The regulations do not *expressly* permit minors to serve as research subjects unless the research involves a condition for which the minor requires treatment. Some have argued that mature minors away from home may serve as research subjects in general, without regard to a presenting health need, *as long as the procedure involves only minimal risk.*[16] A strong argument can be made in support of this position. By defining children, for whom parental permission must be obtained, as those who have "not [yet] attained the legal age for consent to treatments or procedures involved in the research, under applicable law of the jurisdiction in which the research will be conducted,"[17] the regulations imply that all other minors may consent. Accordingly, the regulations can be interpreted to define broadly those minors who may consent independently to serve as research subjects as minors who may legally consent to treatment for the condition involved without regard to whether it is or is not a presenting health need where the research involves only minimal risk.

In Louisiana, for example, where minors may consent to *all* forms of health care with the exception of sterilization, those same minors would apparently be allowed to consent to serve as research subjects generally; so, too, for emancipated and mature minors where permitted by state statute to consent to general health care, as long as the research presented only minimal risk. Indeed, the regulations may include a broader class of exempt minors than intended. It is logical to assume that the regulations were meant to permit minors to consent to research only when: (1) minors present themselves for a treatment, *and* (2) minors are permitted to consent to that type of treatment under state law, *and* (3) the research is directly related to that condition. It seems less certain that the regulations were meant to exempt minors who had achieved a certain status (e.g., emancipated) but were being asked to consent to research unrelated to a presenting health need.

Minor's Assent

The regulations required that investigators obtain the "assent" of children capable of understanding the research—much in the same way that the regulations require the informed consent of an adult. The term "assent," which is defined as the child's affirmative agreement to participate in the research, was chosen to avoid confusion with "consent," which can be given only by those permitted by law to consent to treatment.[18] Whether the assent of children should be required as a part of any research protocol is left to the IRB's discretion, taking into account "the ages, maturity, and psychological state of the children involved. This judgment may be made for all children to be involved in research under a particular protocol, or for each child, as the IRB deems appropriate."[19] The regulations further state that the "[m]ere failure [of a child] to object should not, absent affirmative agreement, be construed as assent."[20]

The minor's assent requirement may be waived under the same circumstances as the requirement of informed consent from adults. Waiver would be permitted where: (1) the risk to the minor is minimal; *and* (2) the waiver will not adversely affect the rights and welfare of the minor; *and* (3) the research cannot be practically carried out without the waiver of the minor's assent; *and* (4) the minor will be provided with pertinent information after participation in the research, if appropriate. The minor's assent may also be waived when "the intervention or procedure involved in the research holds out a prospect of direct benefit that is important to the health or well-being of the [minor] and is available only in the context of the research."[21]

Research Which Involves More Than Minimal Risk

When the risk to the minor is more than minimal, and there is no direct benefit to the minor, additional substantive protections must be observed. First, the risk must be only a "minor increase over minimal risk."[22] The criteria for this determination are not set forth in the regulations, but rather are left to the IRB for determination. Second, the medical procedure must be consistent with those experienced by patients with like disorders.[23] In explaining this requirement, Robert Levine, Professor of Medicine, Yale University School of Medicine, stated that it probably would be appropriate "to invite a child with leukemia who has had several bone marrow examinations to consider having another for research purposes. It should be much more difficult to justify extending a similar invitation to a normal child."[24] Third, the procedure must be "likely to yield generalizable knowledge about the subject's disorder or condition which is of vital importance for the understanding or amelioration of the subject's disorder or condition."[25]

Where the risk to the child is more than minimal, but "holds out the prospect of direct benefit" to the child or may "contribute to the [child's] well being," the IRB must determine that the benefit justifies the risk, and that the "relation of the anticipated benefit to the risk is at least as favorable to the subject as that presented by available alternative approaches."[26]

Conclusion

By requiring that institutions covered by HHS research regulations establish an IRB to monitor compliance with the regulations, the federal government has decentralized the policing of research to the various localities. Also, by implementing regulations which are often vague, or which use expressions that are not defined, the federal government has vested IRBs with significant discretion to accept, reject, or modify research protocols. Indeed, the regulations are often quite paternalistic and reflect the clear belief that IRBs can be expected to protect those who would serve as research subjects. This system has the advantage of permitting easy access by researchers to the IRB (as contrasted, for example, to HHS) and of permitting each IRB to respond to or reflect the unique circumstances of each locale. The system can have the disadvantage of encouraging uneven or inherently conflicting enforcement of the regulations. IRBs may be highly variable in their composition and policy definition. The determinations of IRBs will certainly reflect the debate about whether young people should or should not have the power to consent for themselves prior to majority.

Regardless of the IRB's determination of informed-consent requirements vis-à-vis the federal regulations, state informed-consent law must be observed. Indeed, the regulations state specifically: "The informed consent requirements in these regulations are not intended to preempt any . . . state or local laws which require additional information to be disclosed in order for informed consent to be legally effective."[27] Thus, even if the IRB waives the requirement of informed consent contained in the regulations, the researcher must still comply with state or local informed-consent law. While it is unlikely that state law regarding informed consent would be as rigorous as the federal regulations, there is little question that the state law would require the researcher to make a more complete disclosure than ordinarily required, even if the procedure presents only minimal risk. This would also be true if the procedure, while not classified as research, would be considered innovative or new.

For further clarification, readers with questions regarding research should contact the IRB at the facility where they work or where the contemplated research would take place.

Parental Refusal of Treatment for a Minor Child

What happens when parents refuse to consent for treatment which a physician deems necessary for their minor child? This conflict generally arises in three types of situations. First, consent may be withheld for religious reasons; either the particular procedure itself is unacceptable, as are blood transfusions for members of the Latter-day Saints, or no form of medical treatment is acceptable, as may be the case with Christian Scientists. Second, parents may not wish to impose procedures they deem extraordinary in an attempt to prolong their child's severely compromised life, as may be the case with a markedly defective newborn. Last, standard medical treatments may be rejected in favor of forms which are less traditional or represent outright quackery. The widely heralded case of the child whose parents refused court-ordered chemotherapy for his leukemia and fled with him to Mexico for laetrile treatments is to the point. Actual case examples of each type of parental refusal to consent for treatment are given below.

Religious Objections

Kevin, age fifteen, suffered from extensive neurofibromatosis of his face and neck, which had resulted in severe deformity and caused the right eyelid, cheek, corner of the mouth, and ear to droop badly. Kevin was virtually illiterate, not having attended school because of his appearance. The growth posed no risk to his life, nor had it seriously affected his general health. Kevin's mother, his only parent and a Jehovah's Witness, had no objection to surgery to remove the tumor but refused to consent to blood transfusions on religious grounds.[1]

Disagreement as to Treatment

Joseph, a seven-year-old boy, suffered from Hodgkin's disease. The attending physician recommended that Joseph be seen by an oncologist or hematologist for radiation, and possibly chemotherapy. Joseph's parents rejected the physician's advice and took the boy to Jamaica, where he received nutritional and metabolic therapy. Joseph and his parents then returned to New York, at which time an action for child abuse was brought against the parents by the local child-protection agency. At the court hearing, there was sharp disagreement regarding the adequacy of metabolic therapy. Several physicians testified that the treatment was inadequate and ineffective. Two physicians testified that the treatment was beneficial and effective and did not preclude the use of conventional therapy should Joseph's condition deteriorate beyond control. All agreed to the possibly dangerous side effects of radiation and chemotherapy.[2]

Extraordinary Care

Baby Jane Doe was born with spina bifida and hydrocephalus. Her parents, after consultation with neurological experts, nurses, their religious counselors, and a social worker, elected to adopt a conservative medical course rather than surgery. An attorney, who bore no relation to Baby Jane Doe, sought a court order to force the surgery.[3]

It is not our purpose to debate the ethical dilemmas involved in the preceding instances, substantive though they may be. But it is our intent to clarify a health provider's legal duties if he or she believes the parents' choice will place their child's health in jeopardy. We would point out, however, that not all instances of parental refusal are incompatible with good health care or inconsistent with best medical judgment. Some operations, for example, may be managed adequately without transfusions, even though that might pose an additional risk factor. A physician may well agree with a parent that certain treatments for a severely handicapped infant are indeed unduly heroic and ill-advised.

The physician, confronted with a parent who refuses necessary medical treatment, has two options. Historically, the physician, or the hospital, sought court orders to override the parents' refusal to consent to treatment. While this remains an option, recently there has been some recognition that this role should be exercised by the local child-protective agencies to whom physicians must make reports of medical neglect.

In all states, the law considers the withholding of necessary medical treatment from a child to constitute abuse and/or neglect, and mandates the reporting of all such cases to the designated child-protective agency. It is the role of that agency to investigate these reports and take protective actions if found indicated. This may include the institution of court proceedings against the parents. Under each state's child-protective system, it is the legal duty of the physician to make the required report and cooperate with the agency investigation.

Indeed, in some states, the courts may deem the child-protective agency as the only entity who may properly seek a court order. An example of this occurred in the celebrated "Baby Jane Doe" case in New York State, the facts of which are set forth above. The plaintiff attorney, who bore no relationship to the child, instituted court proceedings on his own initiative to require that the infant receive surgical correction of her spinal defect. He did not file a report with the child-protection agency. The case had a complicated history but eventually was considered by the New

York Court of Appeals, the highest state court. The court, in upholding the parents' treatment decisions, stated:

> [The] primary responsibility for initiating such proceedings [to require medical treatment of the infant] has been assigned by the Legislature to child protective agencies which may file a petition whenever in their own view court proceedings are warranted. *All* other persons and entities may only file a petition if directed to do so by the court [emphasis added].[4]

While it is possible that the court might have been more sympathetic had the petition been filed by a physician rather than a lawyer, it is unlikely that it would have reached a different result. (See the next section of this chapter, "Care of Handicapped Newborns," for a more exhaustive discussion.)

When there is simply no time to utilize the child protective agency system, the physician should independently seek a court order authorizing treatment. A hearing to consider the request may be held in court, in the hospital, or even in the judge's home. Moreover, when there is no time for a hearing, a court order may be obtained and a hearing held later; this can sometimes be done over the telephone. The physician should also remember that emergency treatment may be rendered without parental consent as defined in the section on emergency health care.

Physicians are strongly urged to consider, in advance, whether a parent's refusal to permit a medical procedure (for example, a blood transfusion) might later present a medical emergency, and plan accordingly, thus reducing the risk of having to make difficult decisions under extreme circumstances. A recent case, which did not involve a minor, nevertheless helps illustrate the benefit of advance planning.

Bessie Randolph was admitted to a hospital to undergo her fourth caesarian section and to have a tubal ligation. Prior to surgery, tests revealed that Mrs. Randolph's hemoglobin level was low and that her hematocrit was in the low normal range, indicating borderline anemia. Mrs. Randolph, who was a Jehovah's Witness and unquestionably competent, ordered that she was not to receive blood transfusions even if she hemorrhaged.

During the course of the caesarian section, and through no fault of the physician, there was massive hemorrhaging. The physician initially honored her request not to be transfused. When the loss of blood became severe, however, the physician called hospital counsel, who ordered him to administer blood. Shortly thereafter, Mrs. Randolph went into cardiac arrest and died. At a subsequent trial for malpractice, it was shown that the reason for her death was that, after the physician began transfusing, the rate was inadequate to prevent hypovolemic shock and cardiac arrest.

The court ruled that had the physician honored Mrs. Randolph's request and allowed her to die, he could not have been held liable for damages. But once he assumed the duty to transfuse her, he could be held liable for doing so in a negligent manner. Had the physician sought clarification of his legal obligations prior to the extreme circumstances, which he certainly could have predicted, this case probably never would have arisen; the physician would have been apprised of his legal duties prior to the emergency. Similarly, when a physician treats a minor whose parents have indicated that they would refuse a potentially lifesaving procedure as an incident to that treatment, the physician should seek immediate clarification of his or her legal obligations.[5]

As stated earlier, in situations where a parent's decision regarding the medical care of a child may be detrimental to the child, much of the burden has been removed from the shoulders of the physician and placed instead on those of child-protective agencies. Of course, the reporting physician's opinion about the urgency and seriousness of the situation and the speed with which action must be taken will bear considerable weight in either the agency's or court's decision. Accordingly, the physician's report should detail thoroughly the health needs of the child and the risks entailed if treatment is deferred or withheld.

In reality, the provider's role may extend to that of the child's advocate. Bureaucratic systems sometimes get bogged down, and courts will not always override a parent's refusal, even when medical opinion favors treatment. Sometimes child-protective agencies are so underfunded and short-staffed that they do not take up a case quickly or give it the amount of attention it deserves. Thus the doctor has an ethical duty to follow the case and insure that the protective system is being accountable. Physicians who act as advocates usually will be heard, and their recommendations often have considerable influence.

But what happens when advocacy fails and the court upholds the parents' wish that their child not receive treatment? Do health providers have any further legal duty? Do they have any other recourse? The answer is "no" unless the physician rather than protective agency brought the proceeding. Must physicians abide by the court's decision even if they disagree? The simple answer is "yes." A court's decision is determinative and the physician has no further recourse. Where the court action is brought by child-protective services, the physician has no right of appeal. Where the proceeding is brought directly by the physician or hospital, the right of appeal may exist. Once the appeal route is exhausted, the physician has no further recourse.

Thus cogent testimony in support of treatment during the court hearing will be far more effective than attempting to change a decision once made. It will be helpful to look at some of the issues which appear to influence these decisions. One is the degree of professional concordance over the problem at hand. Considerable support for a ruling in favor of treatment can be gained when there is little professional controversy over the necessity of the treatment in question for saving the life of the child, or, even barring lifesaving situations, for the prevention of significant health harm. But this is not always the case. The determination of what is or is not necessary medical care inevitably involves a certain amount of clinical discretion, and in any given situation, two physicians may disagree.

Indeed this is precisely what happened in the previously cited case of Joseph, the boy with Hodgkin's disease. The court upheld the parents' decision to have their child receive metabolic and nutritional therapy. This case illustrates that when parents can produce expert medical opinion that their choice is a reasonable one—even if one with which the majority of physicians would disagree—a court would be likely to rule in the parents' favor.

Donald Bross, legal consultant to The C. Henry Kempe National Center for the Prevention and Treatment of Child Abuse and Neglect, after reviewing American case law on this topic, identified the following factors which were most likely to affect a court's decision to override parental refusal of treatment for their minor child.[6]

Severity of outcome: Would the failure to treat the child lead to imminent death or substantial and avoidable impairments?

Possibility of deferring treatment: Is the health problem such that treatment could be safely delayed until the child reaches the age of majority, at which time the individual could make his or her own decision?

Probability of successful intervention: Are the chances for success of the proposed treatment relatively high?

Treatment risks: Is there a potential for serious or numerous undesirable side effects from the proposed treatment? Are the risks high relative to benefits?

Quality of life, assuming successful intervention: What will be the quality of life for the child after treatment (as in deciding an appropriate course for a defective newborn)? Note that this factor is very controversial. Indeed, recent federal regulations specifically exclude "quality of life" as a relevant consideration in treatment decisions.

The wishes of an older child: Does the older child or adolescent agree with the parents' position or want the treatment? Note that the wishes of the child, even if the same as the parents, will not always decide the issue. For example, in *Matter of Hamilton*,[7] the court ordered that a twelve-year-old undergo chemotherapy for treatment of Ewing's Sarcoma, even though both the child and the parents opposed the treatment on religious grounds.

Conflicting medical opinion: Is the proposed therapy widely and uniformly accepted as standard medical practice, or are there significant differences of opinion about the probable outcome and/or risk–benefit ratio?

We ourselves would add one more factor to this list.

Basis of parental refusal: Does the reason parents are withholding consent derive from religious beliefs?

Many states grant specific immunity from prosecution for medical neglect to parents who withhold consent for religious reasons or opt for spiritual rather than medical treatment for their child. But many also provide for the courts to order treatment despite such parental opposition. In the case of Kevin, with the disfiguring neurofibromatosis, the court ordered transfusions as might be necessary for surgical correction even over the mother's religious objections.

We wish to emphasize that it is the court's function, not the physician's, to decide when a child shall be treated against parental will. This is true no matter how distressing the decision may be to the physician, and how contrary to his or her professional judgment.

Finally, there need be no concern about liability for making a report of neglect which is later determined to be unfounded or which is not sustained by the court. Every state grants immunity from civil or criminal liability to reporting individuals as long as they acted in good faith.

In summary, a parent who withholds consent for the medical treatment of a minor child can be deemed to have neglected that child. Accordingly, the law requires that this be reported to the local child-protective agency for action. It is the agency, not the health provider, which has the responsibility for evaluating the situation and for taking such steps as are necessary to attempt to override the parental refusal. If persuasion and counseling are unavailing, court action may be necessary. At the same time, the health provider has the ethical duty to provide the agency and the court with as full and detailed a statement as possible setting forth why treatment is necessary and the consequences to the child if treatment is withheld, following the determining guidelines as listed above. Since bureaucratic systems may not always be as responsive as one might wish, the health provider also may have the additional ethical obligation of acting as the patient's advocate in insuring that the child-protective system is properly accountable.

Care of Handicapped Newborns

The medical care of handicapped newborns presents a special set of issues regarding parental refusal of treatment which is in an extreme state of flux. Until recently there was no distinction between these cases and other cases of medical neglect, and the same state laws discussed earlier in this chapter (see "Parental Refusal of Treatment for a Minor Child") applied. Beginning in 1982, however, the federal government, after a series of well-publicized cases regarding the treatment of handicapped newborns, has become increasingly involved in this area and has enacted several sets of regulations which preempt state law and, in essence, set national standards of when parents' decisions regarding treatment of their handicapped infants may be challenged.[1]

On two occasions, prior to the 1985 regulations, the federal government issued regulations on this topic, both of which were struck down by federal courts for highly technical reasons which need not be set forth here.[2] In April 1985 the federal government issued a third set of regulations, based on amendments to the Child Abuse and Neglect Prevention and Treatment Act, the final effect of which is uncertain.[3]

The 1985 regulations require that medically indicated treatment may not be withheld from a handicapped newborn unless (1) the infant is chronically and irreversibly comatose; or (2) the treatment would merely prolong dying, not be effective in ameliorating or correcting all of the infant's life-threatening conditions, or would be futile in terms of survival of the infant; or (3) the treatment would be virtually futile in terms of survival of the infant and the treatment itself under such circumstances would be inhumane.[4] The regulations reject "quality of life" as a consideration in deciding whether to treat a handicapped newborn.[5] Further, the regulations require that each state have procedures within its child-protective system to respond to cases of "medical neglect" of handicapped newborns.

Some have criticized the 1985 regulations as overzealous and too prescriptive in their requirements, thus limiting significantly parental and medical discretion in making treatment decisions for handicapped newborns. A court challenge is almost certain. Providers, confronted with questions in this complex and unsettled area, are urged to consult with appropriate hospital administrative personnel to ascertain what legal obligations, if any, must be met.

Parent–Child Conflict

There are very few reported cases regarding the refusal of a minor to submit to treatment for which the parent has consented, or the application of a minor for treatment to which the parent refuses to consent. We do not speak here about sex-related health care or mental health care. Clearly, a minor may refuse sterilization or an abortion regardless of the parents' wishes, and, under certain circumstances, may refuse mental health care. (For a more exhaustive discussion, see the relevant sections of chapter 3.)

The issue of disagreement between a parent and a minor may

take several forms. It could involve the instance of non-urgent surgery, when the parents refuse to allow transfusion for blood loss on religious grounds, yet the adolescent minor is not of the same persuasion and wishes the added safety factor afforded by transfusion during surgery.

We can also hypothesize a number of situations where parent and adolescent might not agree on the choice between two possible treatment options: when one option may bear fewer risks in relation to survival at the cost of considerable mutilation, while the other would preserve physical integrity at the cost of a somewhat more chancy outcome. A parent might elect amputation for osteogenic sarcoma, while the affected youth might choose regional resection. An adolescent with ulcerative colitis might well prefer frequent colonoscopy to detect malignant degeneration when it occurs, while his or her parents might prefer a total colectomy right away to eliminate any cancer risk.

To be sure, courts would rather not be faced with these types of questions, for they lack the proper analytical tools to resolve them. Historically, courts have opted for the parents' decision over the minor's if at all supportable. For example, in *In re Hudson* (1942),[1] twelve-year-old Patricia suffered from elephantiasis which caused her left arm to be abnormally large and practically useless. Two physicians testified that the condition left her weak and prone to infection, burdened her heart, deformed her chest and spine, and prevented her from leading a normal life; they recommended amputation.[2] Patricia desired the operation, but her mother refused, based on the risk involved, and the fact that the procedure could just as well take place at a later date. The mother's decision was upheld by the Washington Supreme Court, which stated: "[T]he mere fact that the court is convinced of the necessity of subjecting a minor child to a surgical operation will not sustain a court order which deprives a parent of the responsibility and right to decide respecting the welfare of the child."[3]

But, as pointed out by Linda Ewald, Professor of Law, University of Louisville School of Law, courts increasingly may be willing to consider the wishes of minors, especially adolescents. For example, in *In re Green*, the Pennsylvania Supreme Court, while refusing to order treatment of a minor over a parent's objections when the child's life was not in danger, did send the case back to the trial court for a hearing to consider whether the child wished to proceed with treatment. The implication was "that in certain cases the state could intervene to enforce the child's wishes against the parents."[4]

A New York case, *In re Seiferth*, lends support to this contention although the case did not involve a parent–child conflict. In *Seiferth*, child-maltreatment proceedings were instituted against the father of fourteen-year-old Martin, who had a harelip and cleft palate. The father had refused to consent to plastic surgery for Martin, choosing "mental healing by letting 'the forces of the universe work on the body.'"[5] The father, however, stated that he would not oppose the operation if his son wanted it. The children's court had the surgical procedures explained to Martin by practitioners qualified in plastic surgery and orthodontia. Martin was also taken to speech correction school and shown how his speech might improve after surgery. According to the Court of Appeals:

> On February 11, 1954, Martin, his father and attorney met after these demonstrations in Judge Wylegala's chambers. Judge Wylegala wrote in his opinion that Martin "was very much pleased with what was shown him, but had come to the conclusion that he should try for some time longer to close the cleft palate and the split lip himself through 'natural forces.'" After stating that an order for surgery would have been granted without hesitation if this proceeding had been instituted before this child acquired convictions of his own, Judge Wylegala [refused to order treatment].[6]

An intermediate appeals court reversed Judge Wylegala and ordered Martin to submit to surgery. The New York Court of Appeals, however, disagreed with the intermediate appeals court and refused to order that the operation take place. The court stated:

> [W]e are impressed by the circumstances that in order to benefit from the operation upon the cleft palate, it will almost certainly be necessary to enlist Martin's cooperation in developing normal speech patterns through a lengthy course of concentrated speech therapy. It will be almost impossible to secure his cooperation if he continues to believe, as he does now, that it will be necessary "to remedy the surgeon's distortion first and then go back to the primary task of healing the body." This is an aspect of the problem with which petitioner's plastic surgeon did not especially concern himself, for he did not attempt to view the case from the psychological viewpoint of this misguided youth. Upon the other hand, the Children's Court Judge, who saw and heard the witnesses and arranged the conferences for the boy and his father which have been mentioned, appears to have been keenly aware of this aspect of the situation, and to have concluded

> that less would be lost by permitting the lapse of several more years, when the boy may make his own decision to submit to plastic surgery, than might be sacrificed if he were compelled to undergo it now against his sincere and frightened antagonism.[7]

While this case did not involve parent–child conflict, we believe that the court's analysis could also apply to such a situation.

But we suspect that, even today, parent–child conflict would be resolved in favor of the parents if they could make a minimal showing that their particular choice was medically supportable and that they were acting according to their honestly held views of what was in their child's best interests. Indeed, the proper forum for a court to consider parent–child conflict would probably be a child-abuse proceeding, where the wishes of the child are only one of a number of considerations. (See ''Parental Refusal of Treatment'' earlier in this chapter.) In order for a conflict to be resolved in favor of a child, the parents' position would have to be proven to work a very serious detriment to the child's life or health.

Blood Donation

Blood donation is commonly referred to as ''nonbeneficial'' health care. It is an act which does not directly benefit the health of the donor, even though he or she may realize other rewards. It may be emotionally satisfying if the donation is on behalf of a family member in need, or offer financial gain if the blood is sold to a commercial blood bank, or provide the security of a limitless supply of free blood in the future. But these are all secondary matters without specific advantage for the donor's current health needs.

Because the benefit is attenuated, minors who are entitled to consent to health care for other purposes should not be presumed competent to donate blood as well unless specifically permitted by state statute. But a good number of such statutes exist. The minimal degree of medical risk entailed in donation, together with strong societal interest in having adequate supplies of blood on hand, dictate a public policy supporting donation by as many citizens as possible, including older minors.

Almost all statutes limit eligibility to individuals of seventeen years or more, an age at which youths can be generally presumed competent to give an informed consent as well as being all but fully grown with an ample blood volume. Only a few states have less stringent requirements. Oregon allows minors of age sixteen and above to consent, and New Hampshire so permits any married person without regard to age. In California, fifteen- and sixteen-year-olds may donate as long as they have their parents' consent.

The reader will further notice that many statutes do not permit donation by minors until age eighteen. These laws are "throwbacks" to former times, when twenty-one was the age of majority. Nonetheless, they should still be observed.

The decision of an eligible minor to donate blood must be completely voluntary. Acccordingly, most states do not allow financial compensation under any circumstances, lest the lure of money turn volunteerism into exploitation. There are, however, a few exceptions to this rule. In Mississippi, a minor may be compensated without any further qualification. Nebraska and South Carolina allow compensation with parental permission.

In states with no statutes specifically addressing blood donation by minors, young people are not eligible until they reach the designated general age of majority for medical consent in each state.

Organ Donation

The question of whether a minor may serve as an organ donor is a difficult one, raising issues similar to those surrounding the sterilization of incompetents. Not surprisingly, as with sterilization of incompetents, there currently exists conflict among the states on this topic. We anticipate much ferment in this area, not only in the courts, but in the various state legislatures as well. Because the law on this question is in flux, it is not possible to present a state-by-state analysis of organ donation by minors. Rather, we discuss briefly the conflicting judicial decisions and set forth the criteria which a court would most likely consider in deciding whether a minor could serve as a donor.

Cases in which the courts have considered this issue always involve tragic family situations. Often, the minor-donor is profoundly retarded; the would-be recipient sibling is in need of a kidney transplant; and the parents are caught in an emotional tug-of-war. In this highly charged atmosphere, a judge is asked to somehow determine if the donation would be in the best interests of the minor-donor, having due regard primarily for the minor but also for the would-be recipient and the family as a whole. Faced with these facts, courts have issued conflicting decisions. For example, minors have been allowed to donate a kidney in Kentucky, Massachusetts, Texas, and Connecticut,[1] but have been denied permission in Louisiana and Wisconsin.[2]

Courts which have permitted donations have made findings of fact that the procedure would be in the best interests of the minor-donor. By focusing on the relatively slight health risk posed by kidney donations, and the psychological benefit which would accrue to the minor by donating a kidney, some courts have had little trouble in permitting the procedure. The psychological benefits identified have included: the continued emotional bond between the minor and the sibling; the benefit to the minor of knowing that he or she assisted in maintaining the well-being of a sibling; and the benefit to the minor of living in an intact family which has not suffered the loss of a family member. These judicial decisions are based in large part on evidence of the relationship between the minor and the sibling, and on expert psychological opinions on the benefits which the minor would experience.[3]

Courts which have refused permission have looked to different factors. First, they have questioned whether a court has the inherent power to order a minor to serve as a donor, believing that such questions are better left to the legislature. One court, by making an analogy to state law which absolutely prohibited minors, or their parents, from transferring a minor's property, stated that a minor could not serve as a donor without legislative authorization. Second, these courts have put much less stock in the psychological benefits which would accrue to the minor by donating an organ, finding them too speculative a basis upon which to make a decision. Last, the courts have looked to the utter inability of the minor to consent to, or even vaguely understand, just what he or she was being asked to do.[4]

It is impossible to predict how other states will decide these issues, although permitting minors to serve as organ donors under well-defined circumstances seems to be the dominant view. We present below a list of factors which we believe a court might consider in determining this most difficult question.

1. Is there a state statute which would permit the procedure? Without an authorizing statute, a court could find that it lacked the inherent authority to order the procedure.

2. Who would be the recipient? If the donation were not for a sibling or, perhaps, a parent, it is unlikely that a court would permit the procedure to go forward.

3. Does the minor understand and consent to the procedure? A court would be most interested in soliciting the views of the minor when possible. It is unlikely that a court would permit the procedure when a minor presents objections.

4. Assuming that the minor has consented to the procedure, is there evidence of coercion? It seems inherent that a minor asked to donate an organ to save a sibling or parent would feel some coercion. This is a particularly sensitive concern which should be examined carefully and closely.

5. Would the donation present a serious health risk to the minor? The more serious the health risk to the minor, the more unlikely that a court would permit the procedure.

6. Have both parents agreed to allow their child to serve as a donor? Courts would most likely require the consent of both parents.

7. Are there any adult family members who could serve as donors? A court would be reluctant to permit a minor to serve as a donor unless all adult family members had been rejected as incompatible with the recipient. In this regard, a court might also consider whether older minors had been rejected as incompatible.

8. If the minor is handicapped, have all other nonhandicapped family members been rejected as incompatible? A court will extend the most protection to the most vulnerable and will look closely to ascertain that the minor has not been selected as a donor on the basis of a handicap or other "quality of life" issues.

9. What benefits will the minor receive as a result of the donation? Even if the recipient is a sibling or a parent, there still must be a concrete showing that the minor will receive some benefit.

10. What health risks would the recipient face without the donation? It must be shown that the health consequences to the recipient would be dire without the donation.[5]

In no case should a physician permit a minor to serve as a donor without court authorization. At a court hearing to consider such a request, the physician and the family must be prepared to answer satisfactorily the questions set forth above, and even then, authorization is not assured.

CHAPTER 5

Confidentiality and Health Care Records

IN THIS CHAPTER we shall first briefly examine the health record privacy dilemma with particular focus on minors. We shall then turn to discuss recent legislative trends providing new privacy protections. Next we will look at exemptions from these protections and laws governing mandatory information release. Finally, we will suggest ways of managing a minor's record with the view that maintenance of privacy for both minors and parents is not only an ethical duty but also essential for effective care.

The Health Record Privacy Dilemma

Health record privacy never was considered much of a problem before photocopying became widespread, computer data banks commonplace, and third-party interests ubiquitous. Handwritten records remained in the confines of the provider's files. Information requested by others generally had to be culled from the record by the provider directly and conveyed in a report specifically designed for the task. It was easy to discriminate what information should be conveyed from that which was confidential and should be reserved. In any event, once a report reached a third party, it generally simply gathered dust in an archival vault after serving its intended purpose. There was little likelihood of further dissemination or further invasion of privacy.

It should also be kept in mind that even though patient consent for health information release has long been a standard requirement (omitting mandatory release as required by law), this rarely has been fully informed. While well-advised as to who would receive the information and for what purpose, the patient rarely was given full knowledge of exactly what data was being transmitted or what would be done with it once it was sent on. The health record was viewed as the provider's property, with no rights of patient access. Prior to the past decade or so, this posed no serious dilemma in that the then-prevailing system of health information exchange afforded little opportunity for significant abuse.

But when it became possible to photocopy even the most voluminous chart; when this function became widely relegated to record-room clerical staff not in a position to exercise discrimination; when computer technology made data collection, collation, storage, and retrieval a matter of course; and when health care data became increasingly subject to such third-party interests as those of health and life insurers, quality of care–monitoring systems, and epidemiological data gatherers, the prevailing system could no longer adequately protect the patient's own privacy interests.

No limits prevented third-party repositories from sharing stored data with others at will, and this without the patient's knowledge. An individual's health information increasingly became an important element in potentially prejudicial actions and decisions about him or her, and without opportunity for rebuttal. There may not be awareness of the degree of information-sharing, such as a common data bank for more than seven hundred insurance companies, from which, for a modest sum, participants can obtain profiles on any listed individual giving reasons for all past insurance claims and other gathered information. The potential for discrimination in later denial of jobs or of health, life, or automotive insurance is clear.[1]

The Dilemma of Health Record Privacy for Minors

Little distinction has been made between the privacy rights of minors and adults. There has always been the presumption that parents would effectively represent their children's interests. Thus consent for any information release and the exercise of new privacy rights (as discussed below) generally fall to parents, with little attention to potential conflicts of interest, the invasion of the minor's own confidences, or possible future discriminatory consequences. We will only outline some of the problems which may be encountered.[2]

Labeling. Many potentially compromising diagnoses made in childhood often are either conjectural and subsequently disproved or confirmed but then resolved well before adulthood. Yet such information commonly remains in the health record or third-party payor's data banks indefinitely as an established and unremitting fact: unchallenged, uncorrected, and unexpunged. Diagnoses such as possible retardation, learning disability, behavior disorder, drug overdose, seizure disorder, or syphillis, for example, usually have few serious repercussions for the child or adolescent beyond engendering parental distress and securing the care the young person needs, but this does not necessarily carry over into later life, when even a history of these conditions may act in a discriminatory manner through denial of insurance, education, or jobs.

Few parents and providers of child care give thought to these possible long-term outcomes and take preventive or corrective steps. Care must be taken to avoid unintentional labeling in the record, particularly when the information may be sent on to third parties. It is equally important to note clearly when past diagnoses are resolved and of no further health consequence.

Conflict of interests. While parents generally are their minor child's best advocate, this is not always so. In the matter of psychiatric hospitalization, for example, many parents must resort to third-party payors for payment of the bill or else face bankruptcy. In turn, this establishes an outside dossier on the minor, designating him or her to have had at least one episode of emotional disturbance and thereby to be at increased risk for further episodes. The child might be better served by not having such a notation in a repository external to the hospital chart. This is not to suggest that parents should pay out of pocket for illnesses with potentially prejudicial implications for their child, but it illustrates that parents' interests can conflict with those of their child.

Only limited steps can be taken to guard against this dilemma; few parents can bear the burden of hospital costs on their own. Providers, parents, and minors should, however, be aware of their privacy rights and of ways in which they can at least ensure that third-party data bank information is accurate and up to date.

Information confidential to the minor. Adolescents increasingly have options for securing health care on their own consent. The law which permits the minor to consent to a particular form of health care may also forbid disclosure of the record which results. (See "Substance Abuse" and "Sexually Transmitted Diseases" in chapter 3.) But this is not easily enforceable. It is not uncommon for confidential treatment to have taken place in the same facility where minors have also received care to which parents are privy. Consider the following scenario. A sixteen-year-old girl develops diabetes and is cared for at the local hospital. After her discharge, the school requests the mother to arrange for some medical information to be sent to them in order to monitor the girl's health effectively. The mother consents without thinking to mention it to her daughter, and the record room simply photocopies the entire record and forwards it. But neither mother nor daughter is aware that notes pertaining to confidential visits to the hospital's family planning clinic were also included. In this way, the school learns far more about the girl than anyone intended.

Even when the confidentiality of an entire visit is not in question, teenagers frequently tell highly personal matters to their physicians which they wish kept private, but which, because of medical significance, may be noted on the chart for future reference. Thus the record pertaining to a routine health checkup might also contain information about an adolescent's drug experimentation, a negative pregnancy test, or her contraceptive use.

The dilemma about how to preserve the confidentiality of minors, whether related to sensitive information revealed in the course of a nonconfidential visit or to an entire health care transaction obtained on the minor's own consent, represents a major health record privacy problem. Current record-keeping practices simply do not provide for the differential handling of data which is confidential to the adolescent and data which is known by parents. Often it is a parent who consents to information release, and this commonly without the minor's knowledge. Thus the parent does not know everything that might be released (remember, release is rarely fully informed) and the minor is ignorant of the entire process.

A corollary problem results from recent privacy legislation which gives patients the right to have direct access to their own health record. This right is rarely accorded to minors and usually devolves on parents. In many states—but not all—it is quite possible for parents to request and be granted the opportunity to read their minor offspring's entire chart. This could include entries pertaining to confidential treatment, such as abortion, contraception, a sexually transmitted disease, or drug abuse. Laws governing health record privacy have not caught up to those regulating a minor's access to services on his or her own consent, and a serious dichotomy exists.

Parental privacy issues. Health providers record considerable family data when taking care of a child. This information sometimes can be highly confidential for the parents. The record of a behavioral problem in a child, for example, might also make note of such potentially contributing factors as spousal discord, alcoholism, or impending divorce. Assessing an infant at risk for genetic disease when both parents are known to be carriers has sometimes led to the revelation that conception was a matter of infidelity. Infertile parents may have resolved their childlessness through artificial insemination or adoption and may not wish this fact to be known by others.

New Directions in Health Record Privacy Legislation

The rise of consumer-rights activism, growing concepts of a right to privacy, and escalating concern over the compilation of expansive dossiers made possible by computer technology, without the knowledge, much less consent, of the individual concerned, prompted significant legislative change over the last decade or so, including a number of notable shifts relevant to the health care record. While these laws by no means answer all privacy problems and respond to the special interests of minors only to a limited degree, the health care provider should be aware of the general trends.

Federal Privacy Act of 1974

Prompted by concern over expanded and secret federal record-keeping practices in general, the Federal Privacy Act of 1974[1] permits individuals to (1) find out if a given federal agency actually has a dossier about them in their files; (2) gain access to the record and know what is in it; (3) seek correction or expungement of any erroneous data, or, barring this, at least insert a rebuttal statement into the record which must be included in any future record release; and (4) control disclosure to others.

While medical records were not specifically addressed in this Act, subsequent Department of Health and Human Services (HHS) regulations have promulgated a set of rules which govern eligible records; namely, those of any federal institution.[2] Broadly, these rules provide for the following:

1. Omitting disclosure as mandated by law, any release of medical information must be by informed consent. The patient must be advised as to exactly what data will be released, who is to receive it, what will happen to it thereafter, and how long the consent will be in force.

2. Patients have the right to see and read their records on request with one exception. If, in their physicians' judgment, this could be harmful to them, direct access may be denied; but the patient then must be provided the alternative of choosing another individual to view the records instead.

3. Patients also have the right to request expungement or correction of any information in the record they believe erroneous or unfair. This may be denied, but the patient must then be allowed to insert a rebuttal statement into the record which must accompany any information release.

This is the bare outline of rather complex regulations. For example, in addition to legal mandates, there are a number of "need to know" exemptions to the requirement that release be by informed consent. These include release for various administrative functions, third-party payor's accountability audits, and quality-of-care audits.

HHS also promulgated regulations pertaining to minors' health records. Regulations for medical records, which apply to federally owned hospitals, include the following provisions:

1. A minor has the same privacy rights over his or her health record as an adult (when subject to the Federal Privacy Act).

2. A parent who seeks to determine whether a minor has a health record may not be advised whether such exists or not. The parent may, however, designate a third-party health provider to receive the record, if it indeed does exist; this latter individual is to be instructed to consider the consequences to the minor if parents

are apprised of confidential information and act accordingly based on his or her best judgment. In addition, if the minor's whereabouts are known, he or she is to be notified of the parental request.

Family Educational and Privacy Act of 1974

Known as the Buckley Amendment,[3] this act was prompted by growing problems pertaining to information in students' educational records, with numerous instances of information abuse coming to light. Specific provisions, which apply to private schools receiving federal funds, as well as public schools, are as follows:

1. Parents have the right to directly read the educational record of their child under age eighteen in a primary or secondary school which directly or indirectly (as in state block grants) receives federal funds.
2. Parents may seek corrections or expungement of any information they believe incorrect and, if refused, insert a rebuttal statement which must be included any time the educational record is transferred or conveyed to anyone else.
3. Release of information by schools to third parties for any purpose may only be with the parents' informed consent except in specific enumerated circumstances.
4. These rights devolve on the student on reaching his or her eighteenth birthday or on any student in post–secondary school (e.g., college or university) regardless of age. Students less than eighteen and in primary and secondary schools do not have any rights of access of their own, although this Act does not preclude either the state or a local board of education from instituting such provisions.
5. The educational record consists of all documents which affect the student's schooling in any way and are available to any teacher or administrator or other school personnel. The only exceptions are (1) the records of post–secondary school student health services as long as these are kept in strict confidence and not available to others than care providers, and (2) records maintained by teachers for their individual use and not released to any other person. Records of student health services in primary and secondary schools are not addressed and their status is unclear.

6. A student is defined as one who is fully matriculated in the educational institution in question, not just an applicant for admission. Applicant records are not available for parental or student review.

The Buckley Amendment has enjoyed widespread support. Its provisions have been widely implemented; many parents have been made aware of their rights. Unfortunately, because the only sanction against states which have not complied with its provisions is a loss of federal funding, enforcement may be hampered because the penalty simply may be too high a price to pay.

The main significance of this Act for health providers rests in the fact that they are frequent contributors to the educational record and should be aware of the potential for parental review whenever they construct a document to be sent to a school. This would include anything from the evaluation of a child with a learning disability or a behavioral problem manifest in poor school performance to something as simple as a gym excuse.

State Statutes

A detailed analysis of state laws pertaining to health record privacy is beyond the scope of this book in that this is a formidable and lengthy task. Few states have consolidated their relevant laws into a single code. Applicable provisions are often found in isolated sections or subsections of a wide variety of statutes enacted over a number of years. But where a state has a specific provision regarding health record privacy in regard to parental notification, we *have* included a reference in the state-by-state table. Otherwise, we refer readers to their hospital record-room librarians, who often are the best sources of information about health record privacy issues in a given institution. We will, however, review selected prevailing trends.

An increasing number of states allow patients to find out what is in their health care record, although access to mental health records is frequently more restricted. Access varies from direct availability, as in the federal regulations, to having an outside physician chosen by the patient review the record and explain it to him or her. Even when provisions are made for direct access, this may often be withheld if the treating physician believes the patient might be harmed; in this instance, the patient may designate someone else to read it in his or her place. Health providers usually may reserve any personal "working notes" from patient access, directly or indirectly, as long as they are kept separate from the regular record and are not available to anyone else, but they are not immune from subpoena. "Working notes, " however, may *not* be used as an artifice to sequester information that the professional does not wish the patient to see but intends to retain indefinitely.

There has been little substantive change in procedures for a patient's consent to information release. While the legal mandate of informed consent has become widely recognized, implementation nevertheless remains deficient. Patients continue to be largely unaware of the potential for abuse, are eager to have third parties pay their hospital bills, and exercise little discrimination in signing release forms.

Only a handful of states have addressed the health record privacy of minors to any substantive degree. A few prohibit the disclosure to parents of records pertaining to sexually transmitted diseases and/or abortions without the minor's consent. Others prohibit parental access to mental health records. Many of the statutes permitting minors to consent to health care on their own under selected circumstances would not allow record release without the consent of the minor. However, a good number specifically allow physicians to notify parents if notification is deemed in the minor's best interests.

A minor who is entitled to consent to health care is not necessarily entitled to exercise all permissible privacy rights over the record of that transaction. We have already made the distinction between the right to privacy from third-party interventions in health care decisions, on the one hand, and the right to have information about those decisions kept confidential, on the other hand. In law, one does not necessarily follow on the other, and each needs to be dealt with separately.

We would, however, state the principle that preserving the confidentiality of a minor's health record is no less a critical duty than preserving confidentiality in the minor–provider relationship itself, although there is little in the way of guidance that can be afforded the practitioner in the way of specific clarification or direction. Fortunately, in actual practice, irreconcilable privacy conflicts surrounding minors' health records are the exception rather than the rule.

Information Release Without Patient or Parental Consent

A variety of situations exist which permit information release without patient (or parental) consent. Most commonly these have to do with patient care, professional education, hospital administrative functions, peer review mechanisms, and governmental third-party payor audit systems. Public health law, criminal law, and court-ordered releases also occur. There is a duty imposed on all persons involved to protect the patient's privacy and not disseminate the information further. Court proceedings, however, are matters of public record and accessible to the public unless sealed pursuant to statute (for example, family court records) or by an order of the judge.

Information Release Based on a Need to Know

Unfortunately, there is not always unanimity of opinion as to who has a valid "need to know."[1] This has been the subject of considerable debate, and the inability to arrive at any consensus was largely responsible for scuttling federal health record privacy legislation. Presently, a patient's hospital record is generally available to anyone on the staff, due to laxity on intramural privacy protection. There are, however, some governing rules about who should have unrestricted access and who should not.

Patient care. Any information may be shared among those health providers who are responsible for the patient within the treating facility. This does not extend to any other facility, however, unless an emergency exists and the information is important for medical management of the emergency.

Professional education. Information generally may be shared for professional educational purposes within the treating facility. This includes medicine, nursing, psychology, social service, or any other profession involved in patient care. Information only may be disseminated outside the treating facility (as in a published case study) with the patient's consent or in a form precluding possible patient identification.

Administrative functions. Limited amounts of information may be shared with clerical and administrative personnel in the treating facility for purposes of appointments, admissions, discharges, billing, compiling census data, and the like.

Auditing functions. Information may be shared with duly appointed quality-of-care auditors, professional review organizations, and governmental third-party payors.

Research. Information may also be shared without patient consent with qualified personnel for the purpose of conducting scientific research, provided the patient is not identified directly or indirectly in any subsequent report or in any other manner.

Public Health Law

While the specific requirements vary from state to state, public health law commonly requires the reporting of the hospitalization of patients in private and public hospitals, as well as various vital statistics (e.g., births and deaths) and assorted communicable diseases. Other selected diagnoses and procedures, such as abortions, may be required to be reported as well. But strict privacy measures usually are imposed on the collecting agency, particularly for highly sensitive information.

Minors with sexually transmitted diseases may be particularly concerned about their privacy and public health reporting requirements. They should be reassured and advised that all consequent epidemiologic investigations are conducted with strict attention to the confidentiality question and that the information will be handled with tact and discrimination.

Criminal Law

Gunshot and stab wounds and other injuries which are clearly the result of assault often must be reported to the police. But one need not report privileged information about past crimes committed by the patient, including an adolescent's admission that he or she has been dealing in drugs, stole a car, or was involved in gang warfare.

Other Mandatory Information Release

Child abuse. Any health care provider is required to report suspicions of possible child abuse to the proper governmental authority, usually the local child-welfare agency. Most hospital social service workers and/or administrators are familiar with the proper reporting procedure.

Seizure disorder. As adolescents approach driving age, most states require that any histories of seizure disorders be reported to the police, department of motor vehicles (DMV), or other agency. The DMV in any locale will know existing rules. Usually, all patients must be reported, whether under good control or not. Those who have been seizure-free for two or more years will be eligible for a driver's license, even if on medication.

Court subpoena. Any patient's record must be released when subject to court subpoena. While this generally applies only to that record reposited in the treating facility's regular files, confidential files and professional working notes may also be required if their existence is known. Special provisions, however, may apply to records of persons receiving treatment in drug or alcohol abuse programs, and the reader is referred to "Drug and Alcohol Records—Special Privacy Regulations" in the section on substance abuse in chapter 3.

Management of the Health Record

Protection against inadvertent disclosure of information confidential to either patient or parent and the avoidance of persistent labeling of a child in third-party data banks are key responsibilities. Unfortunately, the easy availability of a hospital record to anyone within the treating institution who wants to see it and the the lack of discrimination at the photocopy machine in preparing record copy for submission to third parties can make it difficult to preserve privacy. The responsibility for preserving patient confidentiality largely devolves on providers themselves and what they do with confidential information obtained in trust.

Recording of Confidential Information

The less confidential information recorded in a health record, the fewer opportunities for unintentional and/or harmful disclosure. Health providers have a great tendency to record far more than is needed for either documentation or the provision of care; unnecessary information should not be included in the record. Nor do confidences have to be recorded in explicit detail; a simple generalization may be all that is needed to prompt the provider's memory when the patient next comes in. "Close relationship with boyfriend," for example, may be all that is required for an adolescent in need of sexuality counseling.

Thus the first management recommendation is to record only necessary data, and this in a manner which is specific only to the degree that is necessary for documentation and therapeutic purpose.

Separate Records

While it is impractical to set up a fully operative dual record keeping system, it is not impractical to set up a confidential file to be kept separate and apart from the regular hospital record and under the direct supervision of the provider.[1] This is, of course, routine in psychiatric care. There is no guarantee that such personal, private records may not be subject to mandatory disclosure at some point in time, but there is far less likelihood of inadvertent disclosure, and any required disclosure can be much more discriminating. We encourage the use of a separate confidential file for particularly sensitive information, obtained from either the minor patient or the parent, which needs to be preserved for treatment purposes but which could act to harm either party if openly known. We note, however, that separate records must not be used as a method of shielding records from access, and measures must be taken to assure that such records are known to and made available to the patient or parent upon request, when appropriate.

Third-Party Data

Diagnoses are the pieces of information most likely to be disseminated to third parties for minors—or any one else. They are required by virtually all third-party payors for reimbursement purposes. While professionals themselves usually are the ones to fill out reimbursement forms in office practice situations, this task may be relegated to administrative clerical staff in hospitals and other institutional facilities. Thus it is incumbent on the professional to write notes that clearly distinguish between those diagnoses which are conjectural hypotheses or academic exercises, and hence eliminated, and those which are borne out. In addition, the specific terminology used should be that which is least likely to label the minor or otherwise cause future prejudicial harm. Further, when any conjectural diagnosis is disproved or any existent condition resolved, this too should be clearly noted and any diagnostic list updated to show only what is currently operative.

Another area of unique concern for children and adolescents is health information sent to schools. We have already commented on possibilities for parental review (see the discussion earlier in this chapter of the Family Educational Rights and Privacy Act of 1974). Particular care also needs to be exercised in the construct of evaluations for special school placement or modification of academic programs. As these usually revolve around neurological or psychological problems, the potential for diagnostic labeling is of great concern.

Patient Access

As we have already noted, patients—or parents, in the case of minors—increasingly have the right to gain access to their record or that of their child.[2] In the event of such a request, there will be less distress for both patient and provider if record data are noted, as much as possible, in the patient's own words rather than in technical shorthand. Diagnoses can be handled similarly. "School problem due to learning difficulties" approximates the patient's or parent's own complaint and is far less provocative than "mental retardation." This may not always be possible due to the required use of established diagnostic codes, but utilization of the patient's or parent's own words to the degree possible will make it far less threatening should either elect to read the chart. In any event, should either parent or patient wish to see the record, the provider will be well advised to sit down with the reader and explain each entry and its implications in as candid and as open a manner as possible.[3]

While a patient's right of review may be denied if the physician reasonably believes the risk of harm to the patient by disclosure outweighs the benefits, this option can not be used simply to avoid an awkward situation. In any event, withholding access on the basis of harm would be difficult to justify in the case of parents seeking to read their child's record. The precise legal standing of minors who wish to see their records is uncertain. They have arguable rights of access to data about health care they consented to and received on their own, but probably less standing when they are the beneficiaries of services rendered on the consent of the parents. But we recommend that the desire of an adolescent minor to read his or her record, regardless of legal standing, be respected. It can serve a constructive therapeutic purpose in the service of trust and compliance if the provider will take the time to go over chart entries with the young person and discuss them in understandable terms.

The existence of data confidential to either parents or a minor youth might be sufficient cause to withhold the part of the record pertinent to one party from the direct view of the other. But it may be difficult to explain this to the prospective reader. These are further reasons for exercising care in making record entries. Fortunately, in actual practice, requests by either parents or minor youths to read the minor's record are relatively rare. But for that occasional instance when this does occur, we again reinforce the concept of maintaining confidential information in separate private files, but making sure that such files are known by and available to the patient and other medical staff.

Additional defensive strategy rests in finding out why the individual wishes to see the chart. Usually a parent is dissatisfied with the minor's care or wishes to find out if the adolescent is sexually active. Open discussion with patients or parents and empathy about their distress often eases the situation and allows for a rational discussion. These are the same measures as discussed in fuller detail in the next chapter, "Strategic Issues and Problem Situations."

In summary, maintaining confidentiality of the health care record requires considerable vigilance. The record often contains intimate information of an exceptionally personal and sensitive nature. While this may not seem to be an acute issue for a child, enjoying a protected status in society, such information may return to haunt the individual at some unexpected time in the future. It should never be overlooked that the health record is a permanent document which often is reposited outside the control of either patient or provider, particularly when the patient is a minor. It must also be kept in mind that the confidential information sent to third parties for whatever purpose may well be put to some other use than that which reflects the patient's best interests. Health record privacy can be best assured by careful discrimination on the part of health care professionals themselves in determining what data is written down and the manner in which it is stated.

CHAPTER 6

Strategic Issues and Problem Situations

UP TO THIS POINT we have sought to guide the practitioner in understanding the law and its application, both generally and in specific situations. We now turn from this particular path to suggest a number of preventive and interventive strategies designed to avert or defuse incipient adversarial situations.

By way of overview, these strategies are best implemented when the law is seen as something other than simply an unsavory and threatening intrusion into clinical practice (with the consequence of encouraging practitioners to take an excessively cautious and defensive stance). Even when obtaining parental consent is problematic, the law never intended for minor patients to be subject to greater health harm through treatment denial or excessive delay. Rather the law—and health care law in particular—offers definition of the delicate balance between family, minor, the health care system, and the state, together with direction for positive relationships among parents, patients, and providers.

The implementation of such an affirmative orientation, however, is best based on a basic understanding of the law and its application. Preventive and interventive strategies are most effectively implemented when the professional is reasonably familiar with at least the following issues as fully discussed elsewhere in this book:

1. A basic understanding of legal process, its systematology, and its decision-making methodology.
2. An understanding of the derivations and intent of the law governing parent–minor relationships.
3. Knowledge of the specific legal parameters surrounding commonly encountered health care situations. This might include such issues as the definition of an emergency, requirements for emancipation, the nature of the mature-minor rule, or the meaning of informed consent.

Information Resources

We do not expect that the provider will be confident as to an appropriate course in every case, even if knowledgeable about the issues above. Nor are we, in this book, able to give guidance on every conceivable combination and permutation of problems pertaining to parental consent which may be encountered. Even when we do offer direction, the health provider may wish additional legal counsel—and would be well-advised to seek this in unclear or complex situations. Some, if not all, of the following resources are available in every community. In making a selection, it should be noted that various interpretations of the law are often possible and each of these resources may proffer legitimate interpretations which differ considerably in terms of weighting and argument bias. Knowledge of the direction that such advice might take will be helpful in determining just which sources to use.

Local bar associations. While they do not offer individual counsel, their interpretive papers on particular topics may be helpful. Such papers are excellent sources of information. They usually take an unweighted and unbiased perspective, carefully examining arguments on both sides. Recommended actions usually have high legal credibility and regard.

County and state medical societies. Legal and legislative committees of these organizations commonly have examined regional law on a number of relevant health care subjects; these might include such topics as patient–physician relationships, informed consent, withholding treatment from defective newborns, child abuse, and minors' consent. These interpretations are generally conservative and traditional, with an eye toward protection of the physician.

Special advocacy groups. Many organizations exist at both the local and national level with specific initiatives directed at advocacy for minors. Examples include the American Academy of Pediatrics, Planned Parenthood Federation of America and its affiliates, the Children's Rights Project of the American Civil Liberties Union, and the Children's Defense Fund. These groups tend to weight strongly toward minors' rights, both protective and constitutional. Papers providing legal background, analysis, and/or positions on relevant subjects are frequently available. Some groups are also willing to discuss an individual situation, particularly if it has implications of a class nature.

Hospital and malpractice carrier attorneys. These sources tend to have a conservative perspective that is protective of physicians and hospitals, with a view toward precluding any possibility of litigation even if the provider would be in a highly defensible position. This is one of the few readily available sources of individual counsel on a specific case or on the establishment of institutional policy.

Federal, state, and local funding agencies. Virtually all health care and social welfare programs funded by governmental sources are bound by qualifying rules and regulations which commonly address issues of consent and confidentiality. While these cannot contravene local and federal law, they often provide definitive operational guidelines when the law itself is ambiguous or unclear. Even if guidelines pertaining to minors have not been specifically promulgated, the agency's legal counsel will frequently respond to a provider's inquiries on agency policy.

Practicing attorneys. Probably the most individualized and balanced advice will come from an independent practicing attorney knowledgable about health care and family law. It may be difficult to identify such an individual. Regional law schools, bar associations, and private child-serving or youth-serving agencies all may be able to provide referrals.

General Preventive Strategies

Patient and Family Relationships

Throughout this book we have emphasized a philosophy which places the protection of a minor's health and welfare at the center of concern and as the primary motivation for a chosen course relative to consent and confidentiality. The courts usually are reluctant to gainsay the physician's best judgment when it is exercised on the patient's behalf and for the patient's benefit.

At the same time, no one wishes to prompt an adversarial response on the part of an irate parent or undermine an effective therapeutic relationship. An understanding of the cause of such parental distress will suggest some specific preventive steps. It is the well-established function and societally expected role of parents to be their minor offspring's guardians and protectors in every sense of the world. When some other individual steps in as self-appointed "parental surrogate" and makes health care decisions for a minor without the knowledge and willing concurrence of the actual parents, a consequent hostile reaction is not unusual. Such mothers and fathers understandably feel deprived of their rightful supervisory and decision-making role, and resist having their responsibility as guardians abrogated. They may also feel threatened and angry and respond with retaliatory threats of litigation.

The advance establishment of an open, sharing, and mutually trusting relationship with the family is by far the best method for averting this outcome and achieving parental acceptance of the need of some minors for treatment without parental consent under certain circumstances. The parent who sees the provider as a collaborator in the business of helping the child to grow up well is often willing to share this responsibility and will be far less threatened when not involved in a treatment decision. This understanding is not difficult to achieve when the family is in continuing care and known to the provider over time. If the child is approaching adolescence, anticipatory discussion about teenagers' needs for privacy in some health care matters and the problem many parents have in securing the confidences of their increasingly emancipated offspring is a useful technique in setting the stage.

Even new patients and their families can be introduced to this perspective as a part of an initial orientation. When the provider presents himself or herself as primarily interested in insuring the minor's best health, parents are usually accepting of the minor's occasional need for confidential care. (These remarks will be further expanded in the section called "Preventive Strategies in Special Situations.")

Secondary issues of importance in achieving an optimal relationship with minors and their parents include recognition of the distinction between being an authority and being authoritarian. The provider certainly is an authority in possessing specialized knowledge and skills to be put to the service of the patient. But the authoritarian conveyance of such information in a unilateral manner threatens both the patient's and parents' sense of competence and control. The mutual sharing of problems and potential solutions, coupled with a collaborative approach in selecting and implementing a specific course of action, will be far more productive of trust among all concerned.

Free and full exchange of information is essential. For example, a few moments taken to discuss why minors may need to be seen in confidence (see section entitled "Adolescents and Confidentiality" in this chapter) and to reassure parents that problems in controlling and supervising their teenager are quite normal will be particularly helpful in allaying concern. Similarly, personally contacting parents and providing them with thorough follow-up information after treating a child in an emergency generally will diffuse any tendency for an angry response. In essence, this means that the provider should be able to empathize with the parents' position and sensitively respond while at the same time keeping the minor's health needs paramount.

Advance Policy Determination

Too often the health care provider has given little forethought to treating minors without parental consent until unexpectedly confronted with such a situation. This frequently prompts a hasty and poorly thought out response, often of an unnecessarily conservative nature. Awareness of the legal parameters governing the more commonly encountered situations and the advance establishment of suitable policies and procedures for managing them will be a much more effective course. Child abuse is an example of one such instance which has been widely addressed. Similar guidelines should be developed for such problems as emergency care of minors in the absence of parents, adolescents seeking confidential care, parental refusal of treatment, or the various conflicts which may be encountered in mental health care.

Record Documentation

Even the most defensible therapeutic action may have less legal standing without documentation. The importance of appropriate notations in the health care record cannot be overstated. The record is, after all, the only definitive evidence of the basis of the provider's judgment at the time it was exercised. A few extra moments taken to note the following points is well worth the effort.

Informed consent. Notations should include the scope of information given to parents or minors, including benefits, alternatives, and risks, together with an assessment of the individual's comprehension. A signed consent form which cites these points and indicates that the individual has read them and had them fully explained is important for therapies with significant risk. This applies as much to minors consenting to their own care as to parents acting on their child's behalf.

Emergency care in the absence of parents. Notations should include the nature of the emergency and the potential for health harm which could have accrued if treatment had been delayed until parents could be reached. There need not be certainty as to the actual eventuality of increased harm, only a reasonable possibility. Additional information on any efforts to attempt to involve parents also should be recorded (see the next section, "Preventive Strategies in Special Situations"). This might refer to anything from a discussion with a minor seeking confidential care about possibilities for family communication, to the specific efforts made to reach parents of a small injured child brought to the emergency room by a baby-sitter.

Assessment of the mature minor. When a minor is believed entitled to consent on the basis of his or her maturity, the rationale for such a conclusion should be noted. All that is required from the perspective of the law is that the youth is perceived to be of sufficient maturity and intelligence as to be able to give an informed consent. Additional assessment factors are noted in the next section. It is also wise to note why the minor does not wish parents to know and the nature of efforts made by the provider to encourage parental involvement. Similar but reciprocal statements should be made if the provider judges the minor to be immature and does not believe him or her capable of consent, or if there are other reasons in favor of parental notification against the minor's wishes. The latter case primarily obtains when parental notification is necessary for the minor's protection, apart from the matter of capacity for consent; suicidal ideation or proclamation is the cardinal example.

Emancipated minors. Notation should include the patient's self-reported qualifications. (See chapter 2, which defines various eligibility criteria, such as age, employment, parenthood, and lifestyle.) The law does not require the health provider to have definitive proof; it is only necessary that the minor's representations appear to have been made in good faith and that the provider have no reason to disbelieve them.

While the preceding categories are hardly exhaustive, they do address the more commonly encountered situations as well as offering prototypical record-keeping approaches which may be applied to other situations with appropriate modification. The provider should be able to develop his or her own guidelines for documentation by combining the above with the detailed topical discussions found elsewhere in this book.

A Second Physician's Opinion and the Auditor Witness

Health care providers have sometimes suggested that greater defense against liability will be provided by a second and concurring opinion of another physician. This is not necessarily true, except possibly in cases of major surgical procedures. In fact, the law rarely requires more than a single professional opinion in deciding when to treat a minor in the absence of parental consent. In most instances, the judgment of the treating physician alone is sufficient, and we see no need for a second opinion when the basis for the decision to treat without parental consent is reasonably supported by state law. A second opinion even could be contraindicated when this would detrimentally intrude into the therapeutic relationship, as might well occur with minor adolescents seeking confidential care for highly sensitive health problems.

It also has been suggested that the presence of an "auditor witness" can provide additional legal support. By definition, this is a disinterested third party (not necessarily a professional) who sits in on provider–patient discussions, serving and testifying as a witness to the nature and scope of discussions surrounding, for instance, an informed consent or efforts made in establishing a minor's maturity. With the possible exception of validating telephone consent by parents in emergency situations (see below), the presence of such a third party is always alienating and compromising of the therapeutic relationship. Moreover, such measures have no precedent in statutory or case law and are quite unnecessary.

Preventive Strategies in Special Situations

Emergencies

We shall assume that the condition in question qualifies as an emergency, as defined in chapter 3, and that parents are not at hand. Unless there is compelling reason to the contrary, some effort to contact the parents by telephone should be made, but should not be pursued to the point of detrimental delay in treatment. Reasonable measures would include attempting to telephone one or the other parent at home or at work. If these numbers cannot be identified or if parents are at neither location and their whereabouts are unknown, simple notation of the applicable fact in the patient's record is sufficient documentation.

If there is no telephone in the home, a hand-delivered telegram is an alternative device. In particularly serious situations, requesting the police to go to the home may be desirable. In many respects, the issue here is less legal propriety than the importance of reuniting the child with his or her parents at a time of crisis.

More indirect measures include contacting a family friend, neighbor, or relative as an intermediary (although it should be kept in mind that none of these individuals can give consent except in those states providing for some other adult to temporarily act *in loco parentis* in an emergency when the minor's own parents are unavailable). These alternatives, however, need not be pursued to exhaustion nor beyond an effort which is reasonable. In no instance should they occasion such delay in care as to result in the patient's further harm, physically or psychologically.

When telephone contact is established, discussion pertaining to the child's condition and the obtaining of an informed consent proceeds as if the parties were face to face. In this instance, some institutions have adopted the policy of having a third party (customarily one of the emergency room personnel) listen in on an extension as auditor witness. At some later point, parents should confirm their verbal agreement in writing by signing a suitable consent form.

If emergency care has been rendered without prior parental contact, it is not only legally appropriate but also an integral part of clinical management for the parents to be advised as soon as possible afterward. Depending on the circumstances, this would vary from continued efforts to reach the parents by telephone or telegram to the sending of a note home with the patient or by messenger. Such a note should include the diagnosis, the treatment rendered, additional care requirements, and the name, address, and telephone number of the treating physician, together with a time when he or she can be reached to discuss the problem.

All of the above measures indicate the health provider's clear concern and interest in securing parental involvement, while at the same time optimally protecting the child's health. It is unlikely that an adversarial situation would arise following any emergency handled in this manner. But as a simple precautionary measure, we iterate the importance of documentation in the patient's chart.

Adolescents and Confidentiality

Developmental Issues

During the teenage years, the minor's relationship with his or her parents alters dramatically. Drives for emancipation and identity formation find adolescents spending more of their time apart from parents and less willing to confide in them. This particularly affects those private and personal matters which take place outside the home and within the peer group in that the sharing of such intimacies with a parent inevitably makes them less the teenagers' own, with an implicit—and unacceptable—return to an earlier dependency status.

This need for confidentiality clearly does not apply to those decisions and affairs to which parents are normally privy: for example, academic progress in school, decisions and events affecting the whole family, intrafamily disagreements, and obvious illness. But other problems, particularly those associated with behaviors contrary to parental wishes (for example, sexual intercourse, drug use, or delinquency) or reflecting serious adolescent–parent alienation, are seldom shared. In these circumstances, parental knowledge not only threatens the young person's emergent independence, but also carries the risk of punishment and devaluation, or even outright rejection.

A corollary issue, and an equally inherent part of the separation process, is the need of adolescents to feel in control. Even when health problems are not of a confidential nature, maturing young people frequently resent not being party to decisions that directly affect their lives. Legal issues aside, failure to actively involve teenagers in the informed-consent process commonly results in poor compliance with therapeutic recommendations. There is little that either parents or providers can do if the health problem at hand becomes enmeshed in the dependence–independence struggle, with the patient perceiving acquiescence to the decisions of others as a loss of personal control. The use of force is seldom possible with an adolescent, now equal to parents in physical size; nor are various alternative sanctions effective in dealing with a young person bent on rebellion.

Health providers working with adolescents have long recognized the need of adolescents for both confidentiality and control if their health is to be optimally protected through beneficial services rendered in a timely manner. There also has been a clear shift in societal attitudes toward mature minor youth in granting them the right to act as adults in various situations.

Both of these concepts (child-protective rights and minors' constitutional rights) also have been at the heart of court decisions invalidating legislative efforts to mandate parental consent and/or notification for abortion and, more recently, contraception. In all cases decided to date, even if parental involvement is generally required, there must be some alternative path permitting at least "mature" minors to consent to such services on their own and have confidentiality preserved. The details of such measures are discussed in earlier chapters.

Parent–Provider Relationships

Parents often are reluctant to recognize these developmental and societal trends as they affect adolescents today. But their reality cannot be denied, and an effective strategy on the part of the health provider requires at least some counseling of parents about these matters and the development of a mutual-trust relationship as previously described.

At the same time, a teenager's genuine capacity for independent thought and action should not be denied. There is an inherent duality during the adolescent years: the young person is both a dependent member of the family unit and an increasingly emancipated individual who is moving into the outside world. The respect of confidentiality is something more than a pragmatic response to protective needs; it also conveys recognition of and respect for the young person's emergent autonomy. The ability to respond appropriately to both sides of this duality in an individualized manner, depending on the circumstances at hand, is part of the art of providing care to this age group. Unfortunately this perspective does not easily lend itself to a prescriptive approach, and much depends on the provider's appreciation of all the factors involved and an ability to differentially respond.

When the family is known to the practitioner, it is wise to establish the confidentiality option as a part of the overall family–provider contract. Advance understanding that information revealed by the adolescent, as well as the provision of selected services, may be without parental knowledge—and why—will generally minimize subsequent conflict. In dealing with patients followed since childhood, the previously existent triadic relationship needs to be revised as adolescence approaches and the provider begins to see the teenaged patient alone. For new teenaged patients, such agreement should be part of the introductory orientation at the time of first contact. We again stress the need to be sensitive to the parents' position while at the same time helping them, first, to understand their adolescent's need for separation as a part of psychosocial maturation; and, second, to trust that the provider is just as concerned in insuring the adolescent's growing up well as are the parents themselves.

Assessing a Minor's Maturity

In those instances where the adolescent alone presents to the practitioner or health facility for confidential services and statutes fail to define objective eligibility criteria (e.g., age, emancipation, categorical problem), application of the law depends heavily on the minor's assessed maturity. Admittedly this is largely an abstract process escaping objective measure. But as we have stated more than once, the courts will accept and statutes commonly specify that evaluations based on the physician's best judgment are sufficient. The critical assessment factor is the perceived capacity of the minor to give an informed consent; that is, the capacity to understand the benefits and risks of the proposed therapies and to make a reasoned decision. Points that should be considered—and documented in the record—include the following:

- The patient's apparent level of intelligence.
- The reasonableness of his or her thinking processes.
- A definitive expression of choice (in contrast to a passive nondecision).
- The reasonableness of the patient's therapeutic choice, and his or her expressed reasons for electing it.
- The degree to which this choice assesses benefits and risks in a balanced and appropriate manner.

An obvious corollary question is whether a minor must always be deemed mature in order to give an informed consent. What about the immature or marginally intellectually competent youth? A first consideration is to ensure that what seems to be immaturity or intellectual limitation is real, and that it is not simply the result of the provider's failure to explain benefits and risks in an appropriately comprehensible manner. Second, many relevant statutes permit minors of any age to consent to selected services; here the overriding issue is health protection and the recognition by a state that many minors, regardless of their maturity status, will simply not seek out needed services on their own if parents have to know, much less turn to parents for help in the first place. Finally, careful explanation of benefits and risks to even immature youths or those with limited intelligence can often result in an informed consent. It does not require advanced cognitive function to appreciate the implications of a sore throat, penile discharge, or a fractured ankle, and medical recommendations of low-risk antibiotic treatment in the first two instances and setting the ankle in a cast in the last instance. In many respects there is a middle ground in which maturity or immaturity is less a matter of fact than a condition in the eye of the beholder, depending upon the practitioner's willingness to take time to explain.

Parental Notification

Most laws providing for minors' consent also permit parental notification if the physician believes this to be in the minor's best interests. Consideration of this option is particularly applicable for quite young and immature minors and minors with limited competence.

There also are clear instances in which parents must be notified when substantial risk of personal harm requires protection on a continuing basis. As already noted, suicidal ideation is the cardinal example. Other circumstances, such as an expressed intent to run away or revelations of criminal acts, are more debatable, albeit no less problematic in management. Caution is indicated in making this decision solely on a moral basis. It must always be kept in mind that revelation of confidences without the minor's concurrence seriously risks compromising the patient's trust, and, consequently, the provider's ability to beneficially intervene.

Even when not mandated by circumstances or law, voluntary parental involvement should be encouraged for any minor still living at home when it is reasonable to believe that the parents would be supportive, particularly in the case of very young adolescents. This addresses something more than legal requirements ensuring informed consent; namely, the promotion of intrafamily communication and the enlistment of parental guidance and support. Most of us do benefit from the caring support of some other concerned individual at times of personal crisis and important decision making. Adolescents are not exempt, and it is reasonable to assume that such help for a teenager usually is best provided by his or her family.

While not invariably true, a good number of adolescents seeking confidential care indeed would like their parents to know, but are not sure how to go about telling them. Professional mediation may be quite welcome. In other instances, the adolescent may significantly overestimate the degree of the parents' wrath were they to know. In any event, the parental advisement option needs to be explored in most instances, but never coerced.

There is another category of adolescents with whom it is desirable for parents to be involved, sooner or later, as a necessary component to management. It is difficult to imagine how a pregnant teenager could go to term—if this is her election—and, at the same time, continue to live at home without her family knowing! Similarly, a young person with a drug or alcohol abuse problem can only be effectively treated within a family context. Usually, this reality is appreciated by the adolescent to some degree from the start, but several confidential visits may be necessary to achieve conscious acceptance and evolve a strategy for parental advisement. It is particularly helpful if the provider offers to serve as intermediary; either telling the parents in the minor's absence or being present when the minor tells them. Advance role-playing, with the provider taking the part of mother or father and the patient rehearsing what he or she might say, is another useful technique, often enabling adolescents to tell parents on their own.

Confrontations with Parents

Probably, some of the more uncomfortable moments in a health provider's experience come when parents challenge their adolescents' confidential care. Two general scenarios prevail. The first is parental discovery of confidential services, as, for example, contraceptive supplies in their daughter's bureau drawer. The second is direct parental inquiry as to information revealed during a visit which the parents know has occurred but know nothing else about.

In both instances, it is critical that the provider understand and respond to the parents' concerns. As earlier discussed in detail, loss of control over their offspring's affairs and threats to their self-perception as guardians of his or her welfare are paramount parental fears. It is fatal to respond to their anger with counter-anger or otherwise imply that they have failed in their supervisory, guiding role; this only adds fuel to an adversarial fire. Rather, their legitimate interests in their adolescent's affairs should be acknowledged and supported. At the same time, the difficulty many parents experience in effectively communicating with adolescent offspring can be pointed out. The ability to convey empathy with the parents' position goes a long way toward assuaging their anger.

When the confrontation is prompted by parental discovery of contraceptive pills, or discovery that an abortion was performed or that some other confidential care was provided, little more should be done immediately than hearing out the parents' ire, followed by the proffering of empathy with their distress. No efforts should be made to curb their expression of wrath or to introduce rationality at the initial contact. Rather, ventilation of these feelings should be encouraged, no matter how uncomfortable this may be for the provider or how unjustified parental accusations may seem. Uncountered ventilation left to its own devices frequently abates and gives way to curiosity about what the provider now intends to do. An appointment to discuss the matter face to face should be made for the following day or as soon as possible.

After a twenty-four-hour cooling off period, the situation usually can be rationally discussed. Significant problems in overall parent–adolescent relationships, going well beyond the immediate issue at hand, may well be discovered. When such problems do not exist, most parents will take up their discovery with the adolescent directly and do not need to involve the health provider. When they are unable to talk with their own youngster about their concerns, it fundamentally reflects parental frustration and an inability to effectively or appropriately relate to the adolescent on their own. It is these problems which undoubtedly precipitated the confrontation with the provider. They need to be addressed through acknowledging how hard it is to raise teenagers today and instituting parent-counseling and family-counseling sessions or mental health referral. In this way, the provider responds to the real and underlying issues in a helpful and therapeutic manner.

In the second instance, parents are aware that their adolescent was seen by the provider, but do not know the nature of these transactions, and call in an attempt to discover this. Differing motivations may prompt this step. Examples include parents who are appropriately concerned; those who feel they have a right to such information and do not acknowledge a minor's need for or right to confidential care; or those who have significant problems as discussed above. For the most part, such inquiries are not made in anger; a supplicant attitude is more common. Thus a rational approach can be taken from the beginning. The promise of confidentiality to the adolescent should be upheld and parents so advised, and reasons (as previously discussed) briefly reviewed. Parents should then be strongly encouraged to directly ask their adolescent the questions they now are posing to the provider. Here, too, the provider can offer to be of assistance in promoting such communication (but must never violate the adolescent's trust).

Parenthetically, it is always wise to advise adolescents whose parents are aware of the visit but not its nature (or may become aware through such devices as bills or notices of third-party payments) that their parents may indeed question the purpose of the visit. This minimally gives the patient fair warning if he or she views confidentiality as critical. It provides the option of obtaining care elsewhere under totally private circumstances (as, for example, obtaining contraception at a Planned Parenthood facility) or contending with the issue through some other strategy.

Child Abuse and Neglect

Concern about possible child abuse inevitably places the health care provider in a difficult position. There are no strategies that can ease the duty to report the case to the proper authorities as mandated in every state. Parents have neither rights of consent nor any options for confidentiality.

But certain precepts can at least minimize the inherently adversarial and confrontational nature of this situation. A more constructive approach is forthcoming when the problem is seen as one which is often as distressing for the parents as it is painful for the child, with help needed all around. Most abusing parents do not physically harm or sexually abuse their children with deliberate forethought. Rather, they are unable to contain their own compulsions; or an entire intrafamily psychodynamic structure has gone awry. Some empathy usually can be mounted for such individuals, who all too often were abused in their own childhood and are seriously limited in their capacity for altruistic and effective parenting.

A constructive approach toward a possible abusing parent will incorporate the following measures. They tend to minimize the punitive, accusatory aspects and encourage a positive, problem-solving orientation:

1. The parent accompanying the child should be advised relatively promptly of the physician's concerns (and why), but not in adversarial terms. Child abuse more properly engenders a sense of sadness than rage.

2. The physician should explain that he or she is not making a legal finding that a child is abused, but that the law requires the reporting of any suspected case. There is no option. (Let the law be the scapegoat.)

3. The subsequent process should then be explained. (Child-abuse protocols already exist in most hospital emergency rooms

and acute pediatric care facilities. Private practitioners should inquire of their local child-welfare authorities.) Most importantly, the parent should be helped to understand that even if the suspicion of abuse is confirmed, the primary objective is to rehabilitate, not punish; to provide such supports as will allow the child to remain in the home; or, barring this, to treat the problem and return the child as soon as possible. Criminal prosecution, however, is possible in particularly heinous situations.

4. Ample opportunity should be given for the parents to express their side of the matter and to be heard, even if their account is posed in angry terms. Even if not at fault, it is difficult for anyone to be so accused and not respond defensively. But the provision of "equal time" will be the best method of opening up parents' concerns over loss of control and problems encountered in raising the child, and of motivating them for treatment.

Regardless of other factors, providers must always keep in mind that ultimate disposition of the case is up to the agents of the state, usually a child-welfare agency. Reporting must take place before the child is allowed to leave the treating facility (unless there is no possibility of further harm if discharged home as when the abuse was committed by a baby-sitter who will no longer be used as the child's caretaker). This includes admitting the child to the hospital if disposition cannot immediately be arranged, or even calling in law enforcement officers and forceable restraint if parents threaten to take the child away. Fortunately, matters do not descend to this level in most cases.

Parental Unavailability

On occasion, it is necessary to perform a procedure on a hospitalized child when parents are unavailable for consent. Presuming that all reasonable efforts to contact parents and secure their proper consent have been unavailing, the following options may be invoked.

1. If failure to carry out the procedure would be likely to jeopardize the minor's health significantly in relatively immediate terms, it could be performed under provisions governing emergency care. No parental consent would be required.

2. If the care is not an emergency procedure but is still important to the minor's health, it may be necessary to obtain a court or-

der, or, more reasonably, invoke the resources of the local child protective agency on charges of neglect. (Here the parents would be deemed negligent, and the courts would either take on themselves the responsibility of temporary guardianship for purposes of health care or would appoint the hospital to do so.)

3. If the procedure is wholly elective, legal counsel should be sought.

4. In some instances, a mature minor may be able to consent in the absence of parents. This would most likely apply to procedures with high benefits and low risks. Here again, legal counsel should be sought unless there is specific statutory guidance by either the minor's status and/or the nature of his or her condition.

Summary of General Considerations in Problem Situations

Most of the complex interactions discussed in this chapter occur infrequently, and there is little case law and there are few if any statutes giving direction. But careful analysis of the various issues involved and application of the principles we have outlined throughout this book should offer a reasonable course. Points to be considered include the following:

1. Keep in mind that the courts have always been reluctant to invalidate the physician's best judgment when it is invoked on behalf of a minor and intended to benefit the minor, and when the minor's best interests have been given all due consideration.
2. A well-documented record is the best defense against challenge on any count.
3. Advance planning and negotiation from a therapeutic rather than legal or adversarial position will avoid many unnecessary adversarial situations. The capacity to empathetically respond to the differential concerns, fears, and anxieties of both minors and parents is critical to this end.
4. At least a basic knowledge of the law and its principles will provide some clarity in murky circumstances.
5. When in doubt, consult an attorney.

The Payment Question

When parents consent to the care of a minor child, they are invariably legally responsible for payment of the value of that care. But when the minor alone consents to care, who then is responsible? Can the minor be required to pay? What about the minor's parents? What about governmental or other third-party payors? In this section, we explore the various payment options.

Necessaries

Necessaries is a legal doctrine, deriving from both case and statutory law, which holds that minors can be held legally responsible for certain services and commodities provided to them by third persons, based on the theory that a valid contract is implied.[1] While there is no all-inclusive definition of *necessaries*, they most certainly include food, shelter, clothing, or "other things essential to life and comfort," and those things that enable a minor to live according to the customs of his social position.[2] Needed medical, hospital, and dental care qualify as necessaries.[3] The scope of the doctrine of necessaries varies from state to state and has variable applications depending on the situation at hand.

When a state statute expressly gives the minor the legal capability to consent to treatment, this is tantamount to the capacity to establish a contract. Accordingly, the minor, almost invariably, is liable for the treatment cost. He or she cannot disaffirm the legitimacy of his or her consent to avoid payment for medical care. The law recognizes that when a minor is provided health services according to statutory provisions, he or she also may be held financially accountable for those services. It is unlikely that the parents would be held liable for payment for services to which they did not consent unless they affirmatively agreed to do so.[4] Indeed, many of the state statutes permitting a minor to consent to medical treatment without parental consent specifically relieve the parent of any financial liability. However, enabling laws do not need to include such a disclaimer for parents to still be considered exempt.

But when there is not an applicable statute, we need to look to case law for direction. Generally, the parents of a minor living at home can be held liable for necessary medical services rendered to that minor—even if they have not given their consent—provided they are financially able to do so. This is based, at least in part, on parents' legal obligation to support their children.

There is some conflict among the states as to whether the minor, living with his or her parents, can be held liable for the value of medical services when the parents are financially unable to pay for them. Some states have held that a minor may be held liable, while others hold that the minor may not be held liable for those services unless the parents actually refuse or neglect to provide medical care.

When a minor lives away from his parents' home or is otherwise emancipated and consents to medical services, there is little doubt that the minor is also liable for the costs. But parents *cannot* be held liable for medical services rendered without their consent to an emancipated minor.

The table below, which reflects generalizations based on a survey of American law, may help to clarify this somewhat confusing topic. In each case, assume that the minor has consented to the care in question and the parent has not. Because the doctrine of necessaries is a matter of state law, the law of any particular state may be somewhat different.

	Minor Liable	Parent Liable
State statute permits minor to consent without parental consent	Yes	Unlikely unless parent agrees to pay
Minor lives at home and medical treatment considered necessary	Likely	Yes
Minor lives at home and medical treatment not considered necessary	Likely	Unlikely unless parent agrees to pay
Emancipated minor and nonemergency medical treatment	Yes	Unlikely unless parent agrees to pay
Emancipated minor and emergency medical services	Yes	Unlikely unless parent agrees to pay

In summary, minors consenting to their own health care are, in almost all instances, liable for payment. Under more limited circumstances such as emergency care, parents could also be looked to for payment even if they did not first consent to the treatment.

Of course, the practicality of looking at who is legally liable for payment is seriously in question. Confidentiality is essential for the rendering of some necessary services to minor adolescents; looking to parents to pay the bill, particularly if it is itemized, could well make confidentiality impossible, with the consequent risk of losing the patient from care and compromising health. On the other hand, few adolescents have the wherewithal to pay for health care out of their own pockets and few physicians can be expected to provide subsidized care on a regular basis. This may be a further argument for encouraging teenagers to involve their parents, or, at the least, to work out some alternative financial solution. It is appropriate that young people understand the full range of implications when requesting confidential care and be responsible accordingly. But the dilemma here is that high costs are as much of a barrier to adolescents as confidentiality concerns, and also deter young people from obtaining needed care.

Payment Options

A number of options are available in resolving the payment question, although none, singly or severally, satisfactorily answer all situations. This will probably remain an unresolved issue indefinitely, with no easy solutions. Many cases will have to be dealt with on an individualized basis after weighing all relevant factors.

1. *Independent Access to Public Funds*

(a) Minors who are abandoned, homeless, or adjudged neglected and severed from their families usually become wards of the state and recipients of public assistance benefits, including Medicaid. Of course this category of youth usually is in some form of foster care and the problem of payment for confidential services may not be wholly resolved; a parental figure still remains in the picture in the form of a state-appointed guardian.

(b) Minors who are emancipated by self-proclamation (or so designated by the courts), living on their own but in indigent circumstances, may sometimes qualify for public assistance and Medicaid benefits. For the most part, these youths must qualify as mature minors, capable of living on their own and not in need of foster care. But social service agencies tend to be reluctant to approve this group for benefits, the general perspective being that if a mature minor cannot make it financially on his or her own, he or she should look to families for help rather than the public sector—

alienation, parental rejection, and other such barriers notwithstanding.

(c) A minor who is a single parent and caring for a child often will qualify for Aid to Families With Dependent Children and be eligible for Medicaid as an independent individual. Unfortunately, most states will not make such approval until after the child is born and do not cover pregnancy diagnosis or prenatal care.

2. *Access to Third-party Payors*

(a) Minors who are members of families receiving Medicaid may be able to secure payment on a confidential basis. No head-of-household signature is needed on claim forms. All that is required is knowledge of the Medicaid number and verification that the family is currently approved for benefits. Sometimes this is already known by a health facility where care has been provided previously, the Medicaid number being on file. Sometimes a young person is able to produce a valid identifying card. Problems may be encountered, however, in states requiring Medicaid "stickers" to be attached to claim forms. It may be more difficult for a minor to obtain such stickers from the parent than simply a number. No notice to the family will be sent. Indeed, in a number of states it has been ruled an unconstitutional invasion of privacy for the head of household to be notified of services rendered to any other family members.

(b) Private third party payor family policies generally are not a resource for adolescents' confidential care. Claim forms invariably must be signed by both the policyholder and the minor's legal guardian (usually one and the same person in the form of a parent). In addition, the policyholder is usually notified of claim disposition. Of course, if the adolescent is employed and receives health insurance as a benefit, then he or she exercises all control and the confidentiality question is moot. But this is an uncommon situation.

3. *Prepaid Health Plans*

An increasing number of families are enrolled in prepaid HMOs, in which payment is simply a matter of annual or monthly preset premiums. Thus the possible breach of confidentiality through billing practices is not operative. The only limiting factor is the policy of the plan in regard to adolescents being seen on their own.

4. *Practical Alternatives*

(a) When parents and provider have established an understanding in advance that some care for the adolescent may be on a confidential basis, such a contract can also include payment provisions; e.g., parents agree that they will pay periodic un-itemized bills. If this approach is followed, adolescent patients must accept the reality that they may be confronted by parents in any event, and they should be given the option of seeking health care elsewhere should they wish to avoid this possibility.

(b) When the family is relatively well known to the provider and recognized as giving a fair amount of freedom to their offspring, un-itemized bills can be sent even without prior agreement.

(c) Treatment may be rendered free of charge or at a reduced fee, as has long been customary for indigent patients in general. Adolescents who are entitled to contract (consent) for their own care are acting as independent individuals, and thus should be entitled to financial evaluation on the basis of their resources alone.

(d) In some instances, adolescents themselves are able to pay, particularly if payment is on an installment plan and the services required are not extensive. Many young people have considerable monetary resources at their command and are willing to pay reasonable fees in order to ensure confidentiality.

(e) Referral to low-cost or no-cost facilities may be practical. Various programs are available in the public sector which will provide services to adolescents on a sliding scale, or even free. Such facilities commonly include family planning clinics and adolescent medical clinics: e.g., either free-standing or hospital-based venereal disease clinics and drug or alcohol abuse programs.

APPENDIX

State-by-State Table

NOTE: The following summary of state laws is organized around general headings that include references to specific statutes. In those instances where there is no mention of a particular statute, the reader is advised to check the Index for the location of the related discussion in text.

ALABAMA*

Age of Consent, §22–8–4

The general age of majority is eighteen, but Alabama permits a minor who is fourteen or older, or who has graduated from high school, or who is married, or having been married, is divorced, to consent to any legally authorized medical, dental, health, or mental health service. §22–8–7 explicitly permits a good-faith reliance upon the representation of the minor.

Minor with Other Adult

No specific statute found. Please see the text for discussion of legal principles.

*Code of Alabama, 1975; 1984 Replacement Volume.

Emancipated Minor, §22–8–4

Alabama does not have a "pure" emancipation statute, but its statute on age of consent to health care is very liberal and includes all minors over fourteen years of age. Also see "Age of Consent" above.

Mature Minor

No specific statute found. Please read text for discussion of legal principles. Also see "Age of Consent" above.

Pregnant Minor, §22–8–6

A pregnant minor may consent to pregnancy care.

Minor Parent, §22–8–5

Any minor who has borne a child may give effective consent to medical, dental, health, and mental health services for self and child.

Emergency, §22–8–3

Emergency care permitted when, in the physician's judgment, "an attempt to secure consent would result in delay of treatment which would increase the risk to the minor's life, health or mental health." Statute covers medical, dental, health, or mental health services.

Abortion

No specific statute found. Please read text for discussion of legal principles. Also see "Age of Consent" above.

Contraception

No specific statute found. Please read text for discussion of legal principles. Also see "Age of Consent" above.

Sterilization

No specific statute found. Please read text for discussion of legal principles.

Sexually Transmitted Diseases, §§22–8–6, 22–16–9

Alabama has two laws regarding minors and sexually transmitted diseases. One does not mention any age requirement or notification. The other permits treatment without parental consent if the minor is twelve or over and allows, but does not require, notification to parents.

Substance Abuse, §22–8–6

Alabama permits any minor to consent to treatment to determine the presence of, or to treat, drug dependency or alcohol toxicity.

Mental Health, Inpatient, §22–8–4

See "Age of Consent," above which would apply to inpatient care.

Mental Health, Outpatient, §22–8–4

See "Age of Consent," above, which would apply to outpatient care.

Blood Donation, §26–1–3

Any person who is seventeen years of age or older may donate blood without parental consent.

ALASKA*

Age of Consent, §25.20.010

The general age of majority is eighteen years.

Minor with Other Adult

No specific statute found. Please read text for discussion of legal principles.

Emancipated Minor, §§09.65.100(a) (1), (a)(5), (b)

A minor who is living apart from his or her parents and who is managing his or her own financial affairs, regardless of the source of income, may consent to medical and dental services. Parents are specifically relieved of any financial liability for services rendered to an emancipated minor. Providers may rely in good faith on the representations of the minor. Married minors may, by statute, consent to health care.

Mature Minor

No specific statute found. Please read text for discussion of legal principles.

Pregnant Minor, §09.65.100(a)(4)

A pregnant minor may consent to health care.

*Alaska Statutes, 1962 (1984).

Minor Parent, §09.65.100(a)(3)

A minor parent may consent to care for self and child.

Emergency, §09.65.100(a)(2)

A minor may consent to care for medical and dental services if the parent cannot be contacted, or, if contacted, is unwilling to either grant or withhold consent. When treatment is provided without parental consent and/or notification, the provider "shall counsel the minor keeping in mind not only the valid interests of the minor but also the valid interests of the parent or guardian and the family unit as best the provider presumes them." The reader will note that this statute is more than a simple emergency statute and could authorize care when the parent cannot be contacted or refuses to grant or withhold consent even if an emergency is not presented.

Abortion, §18.16.010

Statute requires a person to be eighteen or married to consent to an abortion. This statute is probably unconstitutional. Please read text for discussion of legal principles.

Contraception

No specific statute found. Please read text for discussion of legal principles.

Sterilization

No specific statute found. Please read text for discussion of legal principles.

Sexually Transmitted Diseases, §09.65.100(4)

Any minor may consent to care for sexually transmitted diseases.

Substance Abuse

No specific statute found. Please read text for discussion of legal principles.

Mental Health, Inpatient, §47.30.670; §47.30.685

A person eighteen and over may consent to inpatient care. A voluntary patient eighteen and over who desires to leave treatment at a facility must submit to the facility a request to leave on a form provided by the facility. Upon completion of the investigation, the patient shall be evaluated immediately in writing and discharged immediately, or be given written notice that involuntary commitment proceedings will be initiated against him. In order to institute such proceedings, a facility may detain the patient for no more than forty-eight hours after receipt of notice of intent to leave.

Mental Health, Outpatient

No specific statute found. Please read text for discussion of legal principles.

Blood Donation

No specific statute found. Please read text for discussion of legal principles.

ARIZONA*

Age of Consent, §36–2271

The general age of consent to health care is eighteen.

Minor with Other Adult, §44–133

When a minor requires emergency medical treatment and the parents or guardian cannot be located after reasonable efforts, then anyone standing *in loco parentis* to the minor may consent to care. See also "Emergency," below. Note that the statute does not cover routine care.

Emancipated Minor, §44–132

"[A]ny emancipated minor or any minor who has contracted a lawful marriage may give consent to the furnishing of hospital, medical and surgical care." Also see text for discussion of when other emancipated minors may consent to treatment.

Mature Minor

No specific statute found. Please read text for discussion of legal principles.

Pregnant Minor

No specific statute found. Please read text for discussion of legal principles.

*Arizona Revised Statues Annotated (1984).

Minor Parent

No specific statute found. Please read text for discussion of legal principles.

Emergency, §36–2271(C)

Emergency care may be provided to a minor without parental consent "when it has been determined by a physician that an emergency exists and that it is necessary to perform such surgical procedures for the treatment of a serious disease, injury or drug abuse, or to save the life of the patient, or when such parent or legal guardian [authorized to consent to care] cannot be located or contacted after reasonably diligent effort." See also "Minor with Other Adult," above.

Abortion, §36–2152

Minors may consent to abortions. For unmarried or unemancipated minors, one parent or legal guardian must be notified at least twenty-four hours prior to initiation of medical procedure. Notification is *not* required if (1) the parent cannot be located; or (2) a superior court determines that the minor is mature enough to make the decision, or that (even if she is immature) her best interests would be served by obtaining an abortion without parental notification; or (3) a physician certifies in writing that there is an emergency need for the abortion.

Contraception

No specific statute found. Please read text for discussion of legal principles.

Sterilization

No specific statute found. Please read text for discussion of legal principles.

Sexually Transmitted Diseases, §44–132.01

Any minor may consent to care for sexually transmitted diseases.

Substance Abuse, §§36–2024, 44–133.01

An alcoholic, including a minor, may apply for evaluation and treatment directly to any approved public or private treatment facility.

Any minor twelve or over found upon diagnosis of a physician to be under the influence of a dangerous drug or narcotic, including withdrawal symptoms, may be treated as an emergency case and is to be regarded as having consented to hospital or medical care needed for treatment.

Mental Health, Inpatient, §36–518(C)

A minor fourteen and over may be admitted to a facility by application signed by the minor and the parent or guardian.

Mental Health, Outpatient

No specific statute found. Please read text for discussion of legal principles.

Blood Donation, §44–134

A person must be eighteen to donate blood.

ARKANSAS*

Age of Consent, §82–363

The general age of consent for medical treatment is eighteen.

Minor with Other Adult, §82–363(e), (h), (i)

An adult may consent for a minor brother or sister. During the absence of a parent, any maternal or paternal grandparent may consent for a minor grandchild. Also, any person standing *in loco parentis*, whether formally or not, may consent for a minor ward. Last, any guardian, conservator, or custodian may consent for a minor ward.

Emancipated Minor, §82–363(f)

Any emancipated minor may consent to medical or surgical treatment, as may a married minor.

Mature Minor, §82–363(g)

"Any unemancipated minor of sufficient intelligence to understand and appreciate the consequences of the proposed surgical or medical treatment or procedures for himself" may provide effective consent.

Pregnant Minor, §82–363(d)

Any female, regardless of age or marital status, may consent to care

*Arkansas Statutes, 1947, Annotated (1983).

given in connection with pregnancy or childbirth except the unnatural interruption of a pregnancy. See "Abortion," below.

Minor Parent, §82–363(b)

Any parent may consent to care for a minor child; however, the father of an illegitimate child cannot consent for said child solely on the basis of parenthood.

Emergency, §82–364

A physician may treat a minor without parental consent where "an emergency exists and there is no one immediately available who is authorized, empowered to or capable of consent. An emergency is defined as a situation wherein, in competent medical judgment, the proposed surgical or medical treatment or procedures are immediately or imminently necessary and any delay occasioned by an attempt to obtain a consent would reasonably be expected to jeopardize the life, health or safety of the person affected, or would reasonably be expected to result in disfigurement or impaired faculties."

Also, treatment is permitted where "an emergency exists, there has been a protest or refusal of consent by a person authorized and empowered to do so, there is no other person immediately available who is authorized, empowered or capable to consent, but there has been a subsequent material and morbid change in the condition of the person affected."

Abortion, §41–2555

This statute has been declared unconstitutional. *Smith* v. *Bentley*, 493 F. Supp. 916 (E.D. Ark. 1980). Please read text for general discussion of constitutional issues.

Contraception, §82–3104(a)

Minors may consent to contraceptive care.

Sterilization, §82–3104(b)

A person must be eighteen or legally married to consent to sterilization.

Sexually Transmitted Diseases, §§82–629, 630, 631

Any minor may consent to treatment for sexually transmitted diseases. The physician may, but is not required to, notify the parents or spouse.

Substance Abuse

No specific statute found. Please read text for discussion of legal principles. Also see "Emancipated Minor," "Mature Minor," "Pregnant Minor," and "Minor Parent," above.

Mental Health, Inpatient

No specific statute found. Please read text for discussion of legal principles. Also see "Emancipated Minor," "Mature Minor," "Pregnant Minor," and "Minor Parent," above.

Mental Health, Outpatient

No specific statute found. Please read text for discussion of legal principles. Also see "Emancipated Minor," "Mature Minor," "Pregnant Minor," and "Minor Parent," above.

Blood Donation, §82–1606

Minors seventeen and over may donate blood to any nonprofit blood bank or duly licensed hospital but may not receive compensation.

CALIFORNIA*

Age of Consent, Civil Code, §25.1

The general age of majority is eighteen.

Minor with Other Adult

No specific statute found. Please read text for discussion of legal principles.

Emancipated Minor, Civil Code, §§34.6, 25.6, 25.7

"A minor fifteen years of age or older who is living separate and apart from his parents . . . whether with or without the consent of a parent . . . and regardless of the duration of such separate residence, and who is managing his own financial affairs, regardless of the source of his income, may give consent" to medical, surgical and dental care. Also, a minor on active duty and married minors may consent to care. The physician, surgeon, or dentist may, but is not required to, notify the parents of the treatment, even over the minor's objection.

*West's Annotated California Codes (1984).

Readers interested in more information should see "Medical Care and the Independent Minor," 10 *Santa Clara Law Review* 334 (1970), and *Carter* v. *Cangello*, 164 Cal. Reporter, 361, 105 Cal. App. 3d 348 (1980).

Mature Minor

No specific statute found. Please read text for discussion of legal principles.

Pregnant Minor, Civil Code, §34.5

A minor may consent to the treatment of pregnancy.

Minor Parent

No specific statute found. Please read text for discussion of legal principles.

Emergency, Business and Professions Code, §2397(a)(3), (c)

A physician may treat a minor without parental consent when he reasonably believes "that a medical procedure should be undertaken immediately and that there [is] insufficient time to obtain the informed consent of a person authorized to give such consent for the patient." Within a medical office an emergency is a situation "requiring immediate services for alleviation of severe pain, or immediate diagnosis and treatment of unforeseeable medical conditions, which, if not immediately diagnosed and treated, would lead to serious disability or death." Within a hospital, an emergency is a situation "requiring immediate services for alleviation of severe pain, or immediate diagnosis and treatment of unforeseeable medical conditions, which, if not immediately diagnosed and treated, would lead to serious disability or death."

Interested readers should see *Wheeler* v. *Barker*, 208 P.2d 68, 92 Cal. 2d 776 (1949), and *Preston* v. *Hubbard*, 196 P.2d 113, 87 Cal. 2d 53 (1948), for a general discussion of physicians' authority to treat patients under emergency circumstances.

Abortion

No specific statute found. *See Ballard* v. *Anderson*, 484 P.2d 1345 (1971), which states that minors may obtain therapeutic abortions under §34.5 without parental consent. See also 57 Op. Att'y Gen. 28. Please read text for discussion of legal principles.

Contraception, Welfare and Institutions Code, §14503, Civil Code, §34.5

Family planning services shall be offered and provided without regard to age.

Sterilization, Welfare and Institutions Code, §14503, Civil Code, §34.5

A person must be eighteen or over to consent to sterilization.

Sexually Transmitted Diseases, Civil Code, §34.7

Minors twelve and over may consent to the furnishing of hospital, medical, and surgical care related to the diagnosis and treatment of any infectious, contagious, communicable, or sexually transmitted disease.

Substance Abuse, Civil Code, §34.10

Minors twelve and over may consent to diagnosis and treatment of alcohol-related and drug-related problems including hospital or medical care or counseling. The treatment plan shall include the parents if appropriate as determined by professional judgment. Attempts to contact parents and the results of such attempts, or reasons why contact is not appropriate, must be set forth in the case file. This statute does not apply to methadone clinics. The parental notification provision may violate federal law. See "Drug and Alcohol Records—Special Privacy Regulations" in chapter 3.

Mental Health, Inpatient

No specific statute found. Please read text for discussion of legal principles.

Mental Health, Outpatient, Civil Code, §25.9

Minors twelve and over may consent to the provision of mental health treatment or counseling on an outpatient basis by any governmental agency; by a person or agency having a contract with a governmental agency to provide such services; by an agency which receives funds from community united funds; by runaway houses and crisis intervention centers; or by any private mental health professional defined by subdivision (d) of §25.9.

The minor must be mature enough to participate intelligently in treatment or counseling and must be in danger of causing serious physical or mental harm to self or others without such treatment or counseling; or the minor must be the victim of alleged incest or abuse.

Consent of the parents is not required, but the professional shall attempt to involve the minor's parents unless such involvement would be inappropriate. The attempts to involve the parents or reasons why that was not appropriate must be documented in the case record. Also, parents are not liable for payment for services in which they did not participate. Finally, this section does not cover convulsive therapy, psychosurgery, or psychotropic drugs.

Blood Donation, Civil Code, §25.5

Minors seventeen and over may donate blood but may not receive compensation. Also, a minor fifteen and over may donate blood with the consent of parents and on the written authorization of a physician and surgeon.

COLORADO*

Age of Consent, §13–22–101

The general age of majority is eighteen.

Minor with Other Adult

No specific statute found. Please read text for discussion of legal principles.

Emancipated Minor, §13–22–103(1), (2)

"[A] minor fifteen years of age or older who is living separate and apart from his . . . parents . . . with or without [parental] consent . . . and is managing his own financial affairs, regardless of the source of his income," may consent to medical and dental treatment. Also, married minors are permitted by statute to consent to health care.

Mature Minor

No specific statute found. Please read text for discussion of legal principles.

Pregnant Minor

No specific statute found. Please read text for discussion of legal principles.

Minor Parent, §13–22–103(3)

A minor may consent for a child, and even though the minor parent is not specifically addressed in the statute, there is no doubt that a minor parent may consent for self.

Emergency, §13–21–108

Colorado has a "Good Samaritan" statute which states that physicians or surgeons, or any other person "who in good faith renders emergency

*Colorado Revised Statutes Annotated (1984).

care or assistance without compensation at the place of an emergency or accident shall not be liable for any civil damages for acts or omissions in good faith." Presumably, omitting to obtain parental consent for the emergency care of a minor could *not* be a basis of civil liability.

Abortion, §18-6-101

This statute has been declared unconstitutional. *Foe* v. *Vanderhoof*, 389 F. Supp. 947 (1975). Please read text for general discussion of constitutional issues.

Contraception, §25-6-102

Contraceptives shall be made available to minors without regard to age.

Sterilization, §25-6-102

A person must be eighteen or have parental or spousal consent for sterilization.

Sexually Transmitted Diseases, §25-4-402 (3), (4)

Any minor may consent to treatment for sexually transmitted diseases. Notification is permitted when a physician believes the patient to be a menace to the health of other persons because of the patient's circumstances or known habits. The physician may, but is not required to, notify a spouse, financee, or parent, or any other person having custody of such minor.

Substance Abuse, §§25-1-302, 13-22-102

An alcoholic, including a minor, may consent to treatment at an approved facility.

A physician may "examine, prescribe for, and treat . . . minor(s) for addiction to or use of drugs."

Mental Health, Inpatient, §27-10-103

Minors fifteen and over may consent to voluntary admission. The professional person rendering mental health services to a minor may, with or without the minor's consent, advise the parent or legal guardian of the minor of the services given or needed.

Mental Health, Outpatient, §27-10-103

Minors fifteen and over may consent to outpatient treatment. Notification to parents is permitted but not required.

Blood Donation, §13–22–104(3)

A person must be eighteen to consent to blood donations.

CONNECTICUT*

Age of Consent, §1–1d

The general age of majority is eighteen.

Minor with Other Adult

No specific statute found. Please read text for discussion of legal principles.

Emancipated Minor, §46b–150d

Connecticut does not have a statute which explicitly permits emancipated minors to consent to medical treatment. A minor may petition for a judicial declaration of emancipation, after which he or she may consent to medical, dental, and psychiatric care. For the minor who has not been judicially emancipated, apply the common law principles discussed in the text. For the reader interested in the judicial emancipation statute, see "Emancipation of Minors," 12 *Connecticut Law Review* 62 (1979). Finally, Connecticut does have a statute which permits married minors to consent to health care.

Mature Minor

No specific statute found. Please read text for discussion of legal principles.

Pregnant Minor

No specific statute found. Please read text for discussion of legal principles.

Minor Parent, §19a–285

Any minor who has borne a child may give consent for self and the child.

Emergency

No specific statute found. Please read text for discussion of legal principles.

*Connecticut General Statutes Annotated (1984).

Abortion

No specific statute found. Please read text for discussion of legal principles.

Contraception

No specific statute found. Please read text for discussion of legal principles.

Sterilization, §45–78(q)

A person must be eighteen in order to consent to sterilization.

Sexually Transmitted Diseases, §19a–216

Any minor may consent to treatment for sexually transmitted diseases. If the minor is twelve or under, notification shall be given to the commissioner of children and youth services or that commissioner's designee.

Substance Abuse, §§17–155t, 19a–382

An alcoholic minor may consent to treatment at a licensed public treatment facility.

A minor may consent to treatment and rehabilitation for drug dependence from a medical practitioner or a hospital. Notification of drug rehabilitation treatment may *not* occur without the minor's consent.

Mental Health, Inpatient, §17–205f

A minor fourteen and over may consent to treatment. The parents must be notified within five days of admission. If a minor requests to leave in writing, the facility shall release the minor or commence commitment proceedings. The hospital may detain the minor for five days to allow for time to file the proceeding.

Mental Health, Outpatient

No specific statute found. Please read text for discussion of legal principles.

Blood Donation, §19a–285a

Persons seventeen and older may consent to donate blood.

DELAWARE*

Age of Consent, T. 1, §701

The general age of majority is eighteen.

Minor with Other Adult

No specific statute found. Please read text for discussion of legal principles.

Emancipated Minor

No specific statute found. Please read text for discussion of legal principles. Also, married minors are permitted by statute to consent to health care.

Mature Minor

No specific statute found. Please read text for discussion of legal principles.

Pregnant Minor, T.13, §708

Minors twelve and over who profess to be pregnant may consent to health care. The physician may, but is not required to, notify parents having primary regard for the interests of the minor. Notice of intent to perform an operation is required.

Minor Parent, T.13, §707(a)(4)

A minor parent may consent for child, and, although not specifically covered by statute, may consent to treatment for self.

Emergency, T.13, §707(a)(5)

Any minor or any person professing to be serving as temporary custodian of the minor at the request of the minor's parent or guardian may consent for the examination and treatment of (1) any laceration, fracture, or other traumatic injury suffered by the minor, or (2) any symptom, disease, or pathology which may, in the judgment of the attending personnel preparing such treatment, if untreated, reasonably be expected to threaten the health or life of the minor; provided, however, that the consent given shall be effective only after reasonable efforts have been made to obtain the consent of the minor's parent or guardian.

*Delaware Code Annotated (1984).

This statute covers any licensed medical, surgical, dental, or osteopathic practitioner or any hospital or public clinic or their agents or employees.

Abortion, T.13, §708(a)

The statute requires persons to be eighteen to consent to an abortion. This statute is probably unconstitutional. Please read text for discussion of constitutional principles.

Contraception

No specific statute found. Please read text for discussion of legal principles.

Sterilization

No specific statute found. Please read text for discussion of legal principles.

Sexually Transmitted Diseases, T.13 §708

Minors twelve and over may consent to care for sexually transmitted diseases. Physicians may, in their sole discretion, notify the parents if they think that notification is in the minor's best interests.

Substance Abuse, T.16, §2210

A minor twelve and over who professes to be an "alcoholic" may consent to treatment at an approved public treatment facility.

No specific drug abuse statute found. Please read text for discussion of legal principles.

Mental Health, Inpatient

No specific statute found. Please read text for discussion of legal principles.

Mental Health, Outpatient

No specific statute found. Please read text for discussion of legal principles.

Blood Donation, T.13, §709

Minors seventeen and over may donate blood to a voluntary and noncompensatory program.

DISTRICT OF COLUMBIA*

Age of Consent, §30–401

The general age of majority is eighteen.

Minor with Other Adult

No specific statute found. Please read text for discussion of legal principles. Also, note that *Bonner* v. *Moran*, 126 F.2d 121 (D.D.C. 1941), case 3 on page 24, occurred in the District of Columbia.

Emancipated Minor

No specific statute found. Please read text for discussion of legal principles.

Mature Minor

No specific statute found. Please read text for discussion of legal principles. Also, note that *Bonner* v. *Moran*, 126 F.2d 121 (D.D.C. 1941), case 4 on pages 44–45, occurred in the District of Columbia.

Pregnant Minor

No specific statute found. Please read text for discussion of legal principles.

Minor Parent

No specific statute found. Please read text for discussion of legal principles.

Emergency

No specific statute found. Please read text for discussion of legal principles.

Abortion

No specific statute found. Please read text for discussion of legal principles.

Contraception

No specific statute found. Please read text for discussion of legal principles.

*District of Columbia Code Annotated, 1981 (1985).

Sterilization

No specific statute found. Please read text for discussion of legal principles.

Sexually Transmitted Diseases, §6–129

Any minor may consent to care for sexually transmitted diseases. The Director of the Department of Health Services or his authorized agent shall ascertain the whereabouts of the parents and notify them of the minor's condition if an examination shows that it is likely that the minor has a sexually transmitted disease. The statute applies to any clinic, hospital, or other facility of the Department of Human Services.

Substance Abuse

No specific statute found. Please read text for discussion of legal principles.

Mental Health, Inpatient

No specific statute found. Please read text for discussion of legal principles.

Mental Health, Outpatient

No specific statute found. Please read text for discussion of legal principles.

Blood Donation

No specific statute found. Please read text for discussion of legal principles.

FLORIDA*

Age of Consent, §743.07

The general age of majority is eighteen.

Minor with Other Adult

No specific statute found. Please read text for discussion of legal principles.

*Florida Statutes Annotated (1985).

Emancipated Minor

No specific statute found. Please read text for discussion of legal principles.

Mature Minor

No specific statute found. Please read text for discussion of legal principles.

Pregnant Minor, §743.065(1)

An unwed pregnant minor may consent to medical care.

Minor Parent, §743.065(2)

A minor parent may consent to care for child, and, although not specifically addressed by statute, may consent to care for self as well.

Emergency, §743.064

A physician or an osteopath may treat any minor who is "injured in an accident or who is suffering from an acute illness, disease, or condition if, within a reasonable degree of medical certainty, delay . . . would endanger the health of the minor."

Consent must be obtained unless the parents cannot be reached immediately by phone or the minor is unable to reveal their identity and the identity is unknown to any person who accompanied the minor to the hospital. Finally, the hospital must document attempts at notification and the nature of the emergency and notify the parents as soon as possible after treatment.

Abortion, §390.001

This statute has been declared unconstitutional in part. *Scheinberg* v. *Smith*, 659 F.2d 476 (1981), rehearing denied, 667 F.2d 93, on remand 550 F. Supp. 1112; *Poe* v. *Gerstein*, 517 F.2d 787 (1975), aff'd 428 U.S. 901. Please read text for general discussion of constitutional principles.

Contraception, §381.382(5)

Nonsurgical family planning may be provided to married or pregnant minors, or with the consent of the parents, or without consent if, in the opinion of the physician, the minor would suffer a health hazard if services were not provided. Also, for discussion of legal principles, please read text, where it is made clear that mature and emancipated minors may consent to contraceptive care.

Sterilization

No specific statute found. Please read text for discussion of legal principles.

Sexually Transmitted Diseases, §384.061

Any minor may consent to care for sexually transmitted diseases. The health service professional must make a sincere attempt to persuade the minor to permit notification of the parents, custodian, or spouse. Notification may occur over the objections of the minor.

Substance Abuse, §§396.082, 397.099

Any person may voluntarily apply for treatment of alcoholism or alcohol abuse, including a minor.

Also, any person, including a minor, may consent to rehabilitative or medical treatment necessary for drug dependency or drug abuse.

Mental Health, Inpatient, §394.465(1)

A minor may be admitted to a facility without parental consent provided there is a hearing to determine the voluntariness of the application.

Mental Health, Outpatient, §394.56(1)

Minors twelve and older may consent to outpatient services provided there is a hearing to determine the voluntariness of the application for services.

Blood Donation, §743.06

Minors seventeen and over may consent to blood donations provided that they are not compensated or that their parents have not specifically objected in writing.

GEORGIA*

Age of Consent, §39–1–1(a)

The general age of majority is eighteen.

Minor with Other Adult, §31–9–2

In the absence of a parent, any adult may consent to medical or surgical treatment for a minor brother or sister. In the absence of a parent, a

*Official Code of Georgia Annotated (1985).

grandparent may consent to medical and surgical treatment for a minor grandchild. Any person temporarily standing *in loco parentis*, whether formally or not, may consent to medical and surgical treatment for the minor. Finally, any guardian may consent to medical or surgical treatment for a ward.

Emancipated Minor

No specific statute found. Please read text for discussion of legal prinicples. Married minors are permitted by statute to consent to health care.

Mature Minor

No specific statute found. Please read text for discussion of legal principles.

Pregnant Minor, §31–9–2(a)(5)

Any female may consent to care in connection with pregnancy or childbirth.

Minor Parent, §31–9–2(a)(2)

A minor parent may consent to care for child, and, although not specifically covered by the statute, may consent to care for self as well.

Emergency, §31–9–3

When, according to competent medical judgment, the treatment or procedure is reasonably necessary, there is no one to consent for the care, and a delay would jeopardize the life or health of the minor or result in disfigurement or impaired faculties, the physician may treat the minor.

Abortion

No specific statute found. Please read text for discussion of legal principles.

Contraception, §31–9–2(a)(5)

Any minor requesting family planning services may receive them.

Sterilization, §31–20–2

Persons eighteen or older may consent to sterilizations. Also, persons less than eighteen may consent to sterilizations if legally married, "provided that a request in writing is made by such person and by his or her spouse if married and such spouse can be found after reasonable effort and provided, further, that prior to or at the time of such request a full and reasonable medical explanation is given by such physician to such person as to the meaning and consequence of such operation."

Sexually Transmitted Diseases, §37–17–7

Minors may consent to treatment for sexually transmitted diseases. The physician may, but is not required to, notify the parents.

Substance Abuse, §§37–8–31, 37–7–8

An alcoholic may apply for voluntary treatment directly to an approved treatment program or facility. If the proposed patient is a minor, the minor, a parent, a legal guardian or other legal representative may make the application.

Minors who are, or profess to be, suffering from drug abuse may consent to medical or surgical care or services related to conditions or illnesses arising out of the drug abuse. Physicians may, but are not obligated to, notify the parents. This notification provision may violate federal law. See "Drug and Alcohol Records—Special Privacy Regulations" in chapter 3.

Mental Health, Inpatient, §37–3–20

A minor twelve and over may consent to admission.

Mental Health, Outpatient

No specific statute found. Please read text for discussion of legal principles.

Blood Donation, §44–5–89

A person seventeen and older may donate blood to any person, firm, association, organization, or public or private agency or corporation. If the minor is from out of state, he or she may donate blood at age seventeen if permitted to do so in his or her home state.

HAWAII*

Age of Consent, §577–1

The general age of consent to medical treatment is eighteen.

*Hawaii Revised Statutes, 1976 (1984).

Minor with Other Adult

No specific statute found. Please read text for discussion of legal principles.

Emancipated Minor

No specific statute found. Please read text for discussion of legal principles. Veterans and married minors are permitted by statute to consent to care.

Mature Minor

No specific statute found. Please read text for discussion of legal principles.

Pregnant Minor, §577A–2,3,4(b)

Minors, ages fourteen to seventeen, may consent to treatment related to pregnancy. Parents may be notified of treatment after consultation with the minor. The physician should also provide individual counseling to open up lines of communication with the parents. The notification provision may be unconstitutional. Also, mature minors less than fourteen can consent to care. Please read text for discussion of legal principles.

Minor Parent

No specific statute found. Please read text for discussion of legal principles.

Emergency

No specific statute found. Please read text for discussion of legal principles.

Abortion

No specific statute found. Please read text for discussion of legal principles.

Contraception, §577A–2,3,4(b)

Minors fourteen through seventeen may consent to family planning services. Providers may, after consultation with the minor, notify parents. Providers shall seek to open up lines of communication between parent and child. Note that to the extent that this statute prohibits emancipated minors or mature minors under fourteen from obtaining contraceptives without parental consent, it is probably unconstitutional. Also, the notification provision is of suspect constitutionality. Please read text for discussion of legal principles.

Sterilization

No specific statute found. Please read text for discussion of legal principles.

Sexually Transmitted Diseases, §577A–1,2,3,4

Minors fourteen and over may consent to treatment for sexually transmitted diseases. The physician may, but is not required to, notify the spouse, parent, or custodian. Also, the physician must counsel the minor and try to open up lines of communication between the parent and child. Notification may occur even over the objections of the minor.

Substance Abuse, §577–26(e),(f)

A minor who is or professes to be suffering from alcohol or drug abuse may consent to treatment. The provider should attempt to open up lines of communication between the minor and parent if this is beneficial to counseling objectives. The statute permits, but does not require, notification of parents. The notification provision may be in violation of federal law. See "Drug and Alcohol Records—Special Privacy Regulations" in chapter 3.

Mental Health, Inpatient, §334–60.1

A person must be eighteen to consent to admission.

Mental Health, Outpatient

No specific statute found. Please read text for discussion of legal principles.

Blood Donation

No specific statute found. Please read text for discussion of legal principles.

IDAHO*

Age of Consent, §32–101(1),(2)

The general age of majority is eighteen.

*Idaho Code (1985).

Minor with Other Adult, §39–4303(b)

"If no parent, spouse, or legal guardian is readily available to do so, the consent [for the furnishing of hospital, medical, dental, or surgical care, treatment, or procedures] may be given by any competent relative representing himself or herself to be an appropriate responsible person to act under the circumstances; and, in the case of a never married minor . . . by any other competent individual representing himself or herself to be responsible for the health care of such person."

Emancipated Minor

No specific statute found. Please read text for discussion of legal principles. Also, see "Mature Minor," below.

Mature Minor, §39–4302

Idaho has a statute which states the following: "Any person of ordinary intelligence and awareness sufficient for him or her generally to comprehend the need for, the nature of and the significant risks ordinarily inherent in any contemplated hospital, medical, dental or surgical care, treatment or procedure is competent to consent thereto on his own behalf. Any physician, dentist, hospital or other duly authorized person may provide such health care and services in reliance upon such a consent if the consenting person appears to the physician or dentist securing the consent to possess such requisite intelligence and awareness at the time of giving it." While this would appear to include mature minors, the statute later differentiates between minors and adults. Thus, the effect of the section quoted above is unclear.

Pregnant Minor

No specific statute found. Please read text for discussion of legal principles. See also "Mature Minor," above.

Minor Parent

No specific statute found. Please read text for discussion of legal principles. See also "Mature Minor," above.

Emergency, §39–4303(c)

When no person is readily available and willing to give or refuse consent, the minor may be treated when "in the judgment of the attending physician or dentist [the minor] presents a medical emergency or there is substantial likelihood of his or her life or health being seriously endangered by withholding or delay in the rendering of such hospital, medical, dental or surgical care."

Abortion, §18–609(6)

Minors may consent to abortions, but the statute requires notification of parents for unmarried or unemancipated minors. This statute is probably unconstitutional as applied to mature minors. In addition, there is a substantial question whether the statute is constitutional as applied to immature minors, because it does not provide an alternate procedure for determination of whether notification is in the best interests of the minor. Please read text for discussion of legal principles.

Contraception, §18–603

Any person who is sufficiently intelligent and mature in the health care provider's opinion can be examined and obtain contraceptives and information on contraceptives.

Sterilization

No specific statute found. Please read text for discussion of legal principles.

Sexually Transmitted Diseases, §39–3801

Any minor fourteen or older may consent to treatment of sexually transmitted diseases.

Substance Abuse, §37–3102, §39–307

Any person may request treatment or rehabilitation for addiction to or dependency on drugs. If the person is sixteen or older, the fact that he or she sought or received treatment may not be disclosed without the minor's consent. Also, the minor must be counseled about the benefits of involving parents in treatment. To the extent that the statute permits notification of treatment to parents of minors less than sixteen, it may be in violation of federal law. See "Drug and Alcohol Records—Special Privacy Regulations" in chapter 3.

Also, any alcoholic may apply for treatment to any approved public treatment facility.

Mental Health, Inpatient, §§66–318, 320

Any emancipated minor may consent to admission. Also, unemancipated minors fourteen to seventeen may consent to admission and the facility director must notify the parent. The minor may request release in writing, but if the minor, by reason of age, was admitted on the application of another person, his or her release, prior to becoming sixteen years of age, may be conditioned upon the consent of a parent or guardian.

Mental Health, Outpatient

No specific statute found. Pleaes read text for discussion of legal principles. Also, see "Mature Minor," above.

Blood Donation, §39–3701

Minors seventeen and over may donate blood to voluntary noncompensatory programs.

ILLINOIS*

Age of Consent, C. 111, §4501

Persons may consent to medical treatment at eighteen years of age.

Minor with Other Adult

No specific statute found. Please read text for discussion of legal principles.

Emancipated Minor

No specific medical consent statute found. Please read text for discussion of legal principles. Also, married minors are permitted by statute to consent to health care. Last, Illinois has a statutory procedure whereby a minor may obtain a judicial declaration of emancipation. C. 40, §§2201–2211.

Mature Minor

No specific statute found. Please read text for discussion of legal principles.

Pregnant Minor, C. 111, §4501

A pregnant minor may consent to medical and surgical procedures.

Minor Parent, C. 111, §4502

A minor parent may consent to health care of child. Also, although not specifically covered by the statute, a minor parent may consent to treatment for self.

Emergency, C. 111, §4503

"Where a hospital or a physician, licensed to practice medicine or sur-

*Smith–Hurd Illinois Statutes Annotated (1985).

gery, renders emergency treatment or first-aid or a licensed dentist renders emergency dental treatment to a minor, consent of the minor's parent or legal guardian need not be obtained if, in the sole opinion of the physician, dentist or hospital, the obtaining of consent is not reasonably feasible under the circumstances without adversely affecting the condition of such minor's health."

Abortion, C. 38, §§81–61 through §81–70

Minors may consent to abortions. The statute requires advance notice of twenty-four hours to parents of unemancipated minors. If the minor objects to notification, she may file a petition for waiver in the circuit court. Notification shall be waived if the minor is mature and well-informed enough to make the abortion decision or the waiver would be in her best interests. Notification is not required under emergency circumstances, which must be documented in the record, or if the parents have already been notified, or if the parents accompany the minor to the place where the abortion is to be performed, or submit a notarized statement indicating that they have been notified.

NOTE: The twenty-four hour waiting period was declared unconstitutional, and the entire Parental Notice of Abortion Act, described above, was enjoined until the Illinois Supreme Court promulgates rules which assure the expeditious and confidential dispositions of petitions for waivers of parental notification made to the circuit courts. *Zbaraz* v. *Hartigan*, 763 F.2d 1532 (7th Cir. 1985). This case is on appeal to the U.S. Supreme Court.

Contraception, C. 111½, §4651

Consent of parents is required unless the minor is married, or a parent, or pregnant, or a serious health hazard would be created without such services, or the minor is referred by a physician, clergyman, or a planned parenthood agency.

To the extent that this statute could be read to limit the right of a mature or emancipated minor to consent to the receipt of contraceptive care, it is unconstitutional.

Sterilization

No specific statute found. Please read text for discussion of legal principles.

Sexually Transmitted Diseases, C. 111, §§4504, 4505

Minors twelve and over may consent to treatment for sexually transmitted diseases. The provider may, but is not required to, notify the parents. Also the provider, with the consent of the minor, must make reasonable efforts to involve the family if that is not detrimental to the minor's progress and care. In addition, the provider must make reasonable efforts to assist the minor to accept family involvement.

Substance Abuse, C. 111, §§4504, 4505

Minors twelve and over who suffer from alcohol abuse or from the use of depressant or stimulant drugs or narcotics may consent to treatment and counseling. Reasonable efforts must be made to involve the minor's family in treatment and to assist the minor to accept family involvement, if these efforts are not detrimental to the minor's progress and care.

When a minor is treated for drug or alcohol abuse, the provider may, but is not required to, notify the parents. This provision may violate federal law. See "Drug and Alcohol Records—Special Privacy Regulations" in chapter 3.

When the minor is treated for alcohol abuse, notification of parents must occur after the second visit unless this would jeopardize treatment, but in any event notification must occur within three months of the institution of treatment. This provision may also violate federal law. See "Drug and Alcohol Records—Special Privacy Regulations" in chapter 3.

Mental Health, Inpatient, C. 91½, §§3–502, 504

Minors sixteen and over may consent to admission. The minor's parents or guardian, or a person standing *in loco parentis*, shall be immediately informed of the admission. In emergencies, an interested person age eighteen or older may consent to admission of a minor if the parents cannot be located or refuse to consent.

Mental Health, Outpatient, C. 91½, §3–501

Minors fourteen and over may consent to outpatient treatment. The consent is limited to five sessions lasting not more than forty-five minutes each until the parent, guardian, or person standing *in loco parentis* consents.

The minor's parents, guardian, or person standing *in loco parentis* shall not be informed of outpatient counseling or psychotherapy without the consent of the minor unless the facility director believes such disclosure is necessary. If the facility director intends to disclose the fact of counseling or psychotherapy, the minor shall be so informed. However, until the parents are notified, counseling must be limited to five sessions of forty-five minutes each.

Finally, the minor's parent or guardian, or a person standing *in loco parentis*, shall not be liable for the costs of outpatient counseling or psychotherapy received without his or her consent.

Blood Donation, C. 111½, §600

Minors seventeen and over may consent to donating blood, but the decision must be completely voluntary.

INDIANA*

Age of Consent, §16–8–3–1

Persons may consent to medical treatment at age eighteen.

Minor with Other Adult, §16–8–3–1

If a minor has no parents, consent to medical treatment may be provided by the minor's legal guardian, or, if the minor is neglected, by the agency of which he was made a ward by the juvenile court.

For situations not covered by this statute, please read the text for discussion of legal principles.

Emancipated Minor, §16–8–4–1, §16–8–3–1

Emancipated and married minors may consent to medical treatment.

Mature Minor

No specific statute found. Please read text for discussion of legal principles. Also, interested readers should see 1948 Op. Att'y Gen. 289, in which the Attorney General stated: "In some instances, even though the exigencies of a situation do not demand an immediate operation, i.e. where there is no imminent peril to life, a surgeon may operate [on] a mature youth, if his consent has been given, and ostensibly the parent has consented, although no express consent of the parent has been granted, and no liability will result."

Pregnant Minor

No specific statute found. Please read text for discussion of legal principles.

Minor Parent, §16–8–4–2

Any person who is the parent of a child may consent to care for self and the child.

*Burns Indiana Statutes (1984).

Emergency, §16–8–3–2

Physicians may provide emergency treatment to minors without parental consent. Although the term "emergency" is not defined in the statute, the Attorney General has stated that it is used in its common meaning and would include procedures necessary for preservation of life or to prevent further aggravated physical injury. See 1948 Op. Att'y Gen. 289.

Abortion, §35–1–58.5–2.5

A minor must be eighteen to consent to an abortion unless emancipated. An unemancipated minor who objects to the parental consent requirement may petition the juvenile court for a waiver of that requirement. The court must waive the requirement if it finds that the minor is mature enough to make the abortion decision or that the abortion would be in her best interests. A physician who feels that the requirement of parental consent would have an adverse affect on the minor may also petition the juvenile court for a waiver. Last, consent is not required under emergency circumstances where the continued pregnancy provides an immediate threat and grave risk to the life or health of the minor.

Contraception

No specific statute found. Please read text for discussion of legal principles.

Sterilization

No specific statute found. Please read text for discussion of legal principles.

Sexually Transmitted Diseases, §16–8–5–1

Any minor may consent to medical treatment for sexually transmitted diseases.

Substance Abuse, §16–13–6.1–23

Any minor may consent to treatment for alcoholism, or alcohol or drug abuse, from a facility approved by the Division of Addiction Services. Notification of the parents is left to the discretion of the provider. The notification provision may violate federal law. See "Drug and Alcohol Records—Special Privacy Regulations" in chapter 3.

Mental Health, Inpatient, §16–14–9.1–2

A person must be eighteen to consent to admission.

Mental Health, Outpatient

No specific statute found. Please read text for discussion of legal principles.

Blood Donation, §16–8–2–1

Seventeen-year-olds may consent to voluntary and noncompensatory programs.

IOWA*

Age of Consent, §599.1

The general age of majority is eighteen.

Minor with Other Adult

No specific statute found. Please read text for discussion of legal principles.

Emancipated Minor

No specific statute found. Please read text for discussion of legal principles. A married minor, by statute, may consent to health care.

Mature Minor

No specific statute found. Please read text for discussion of legal principles.

Pregnant Minor

No specific statute found. Please read text for discussion of legal principles.

Minor Parent

No specific statute found. Please read text for discussion of legal principles.

Emergency, §147A.10(2)

Iowa does not have a pure emergency statute but does have a statute which releases physicians, a physician's designees, certified advanced

*Iowa Code Annotated (1985).

EMTs or paramedics from liability for failure to obtain consent under emergency circumstances where there is no one "reasonably available who is legally authorized to consent to the providing of such care."

Also, case 3 in Chapter 3, *Jackovach* v. *Yocum*, 237 N. W. 444 (Iowa 1931), is from Iowa and is discussed on page 52.

Abortion

No specific statute found. Please read text for discussion of legal principles. Interested readers should also refer to 1976 Op. Att'y Gen. 9272 (7/15/76), in which he declared that the state may not impose blanket provisions requiring parental consent for abortions for unmarried minors during the first twelve weeks of pregnancy.

Contraception

No specific statute found. Please read text for discussion of legal principles.

Sterilization

No specific statute found. Please read text for discussion of legal principles.

Sexually Transmitted Diseases, §140.9

Minors may consent to treatment for sexually transmitted diseases.

Substance Abuse, §125.33

Any minor may consent to services for abuse of chemical substances. Services rendered may not be reported to or discussed with the parents unless the minor consents.

Mental Health, Inpatient, §229.2

A person must be eighteen to consent to admission. Upon receipt of a parent's application for voluntary admission of a minor, the chief medical officer shall provide separate prescreening interviews and consultations with the parent and the minor to assess the family environment and the appropriateness of the application for admission. If the chief medical officer of the hospital to which the application is made determines that the admission is appropriate but the minor objects, the parent must petition the juvenile court for approval before the minor is actually admitted.

Mental Health, Outpatient

No specific statute found. Please read text for discussion of legal principles.

Blood Donation, §599.6

Persons seventeen or older may donate blood to voluntary and noncompensatory programs.

KANSAS*

Age of Consent, §§38–101, 38–123b

The general age of majority is eighteen. However, a minor sixteen and over may consent to medical treatment, including hospital and surgical treatment, if the parent is not immediately available.

Minor with Other Adult

No specific statute found. Please read text for discussion of legal principles.

Emancipated Minor

No specific medical consent statute found. Please read text for discussion of legal principles. Also, see "Age of Consent," above.

Mature Minor

No specific statute found. Please read text for discussion of legal principles. Also, see *Younts* v. *St. Francis Hospital*, 469 P.2d 330 (1970)—case 2 on page 44—where the Supreme Court of Kansas specifically recognized the mature-minor doctrine when a seventeen-year-old was of sufficient age and maturity to understand the nature and consequences of a minor surgical procedure. Also, see "Age of Consent," above.

Pregnant Minor, §38–123

A pregnant minor may consent to pregnancy treatment when no parent is available. The term "available" is not defined in the statute, but it is clear that regardless of this statute, a pregnant minor may so consent without parental consent. Please read text for discussion of legal principles.

*Kansas Statutes (1984).

Minor Parent, §38–122

A minor may consent to care for child, and, although not specifically covered by the statute, may consent for self as well.

Emergency, §65–2891

Any health care provider may provide emergency services to a minor. The statute covers any health care provider licensed to practice in any branch of healing arts.

Abortion, §38–123

The consent of the parent is not required where the parent is not available. The term "available" is not defined in the statute. This statute is unconstitutional to the extent that it would prevent mature or emancipated minors from obtaining abortions without parental consent, or to the extent that it does not provide an alternate procedure for a determination that the abortion may be in the best interests of an immature minor, thus not requiring parental consent. Please read text for discussion of legal principles.

Contraception, §23–501

This statute would require parental consent for services from state-established family planning centers unless the patient is eighteen. The statute is probably unconstitutional to the extent that it prevents mature and emancipated minors from obtaining contraceptives without parental consent. Please see text for discussion of legal principles.

Sterilization

No specific statute found. Please read text for discussion of legal principles.

Sexually Transmitted Diseases, §65–2892

Any minor may consent to treatment for sexually transmitted diseases. The parent or custodian may be notified in accord with the provider's opinion of what will be most beneficial to the minor.

Substance Abuse, §65–2892a

No specific statute found regarding alcohol abuse. Please read text for discussion of legal principles.

Any minor may be treated for drug abuse, misuse, or addiction.

Mental Health, Inpatient, §59–2905

Minors fourteen and over may consent to admission. The minor's parents must be promptly notified of such admission. Also, the minor who applied for admission may request release on his or her own behalf and the parents must be notified promptly.

Mental Health, Outpatient

No specific statute found. Please read text for discussion of legal principles. Also, see "Age of Consent," above.

Blood Donation, §38–123a

Minors seventeen and over may donate blood if done voluntarily and without compensation.

KENTUCKY*

Age of Consent, §2.015

The general age of majority is eighteen. For purposes of the care and treatment of the handicapped, twenty-one years is the age of majority.

Minor with Other Adult

No specific statute found. Please read text for discussion of legal principles.

Emancipated Minor, §214.185

Any emancipated minor may consent to medical treatment. The health service provider may notify the minor's parents if notification would benefit the minor.

Mature Minor

No specific statute found. Please read text for discussion of legal principles.

Pregnant Minor, §214.185

A minor may consent to pregnancy care. This statute would allow notification of the parent if deemed a benefit to the minor. This notification provision may be of questionable constitutionality. Please read text for discussion of legal principles.

*Kentucky Revised Statutes (1984).

Minor Parent, §214.185

A minor parent may consent to treatment for self and child. Notification of the minor's parents is permitted if it would benefit the minor.

Emergency, §214.185

Medical, dental, or other health services may be rendered to a minor when "in the professional's judgment, the risk to the minor's life or health is of such a nature that treatment should be given without delay" and "the requirement of consent would result in a delay or denial of treatment."

The health service provider may look to the parent for payment if the services were essential to preserve the health of the minor. Notification is permitted if it would benefit the health of the minor.

Abortion, §311.732

A minor must be eighteen to consent to an abortion unless emancipated. The unemancipated minor may seek to have the requirement of parental consent waived by petitioning the circuit court. The court must waive the requirement if it finds that the minor is sufficiently mature or competent to give informed consent to the abortion. If the minor is too immature to consent to the abortion, the court may permit the procedure to go forward if it is in the minor's best interests, after consulting with the parents of the minor if reasonably possible. The court, however, does not have to consult with the parents if that would not be in the minor's best interests.

Contraception, §214.185

A minor may consent to contraceptive care. This does not include sterilization.

Sterilization, §212.345

Adult parents must consent for nontherapeutic sterilizations of unmarried children.

Sexually Transmitted Diseases, §214.185

Any minor may consent to treatment for sexually transmitted diseases. The provider may, but is not required to, notify parents if, in the provider's judgment, notification would benefit the health of the minor.

Substance Abuse, §§214.185, 222.440

A minor who suffers from alcoholism or who is under the influence of alcohol may be treated.

A minor may be treated by a physician for drug abuse or addiction or for being under the influence of drugs.

In both cases, the provider may notify the parents, if, in the provider's judgment, that would benefit the health of the minor. These notification provisions may violate federal law. See "Drug and Alcohol Records—Special Privacy Regulations" in chapter 3.

Mental Health, Inpatient, §202A.021

Minors fourteen and over may consent to admission with the concurrence of the treating or admitting physician. The parents must be immediately informed of the admission.

Mental Health, Outpatient

No specific statute found. Please read text for discussion of legal principles.

Blood Donation

No specific statute found. Please read text for discussion of legal principles.

LOUISIANA*

Age of Consent, R.S. 40:1095

Any minor "who is or believes himself to be afflicted with an illness or disease" may consent to medical treatment. The health service provider may, but is not required to, notify the parents about the treatment.

Minor with Other Adult, R.S. 40:1299.53

In the absence of a parent, any adult may consent to medical or surgical treatment for a minor brother or sister.

In the absence of a parent, any grandparent may consent to medical or surgical treatment for a minor grandchild.

Any person temporarily standing *in loco parentis*, whether formally serving or not, may consent to medical or surgical care for a ward.

Emancipated Minor

No specific statute found. But see "Age of Consent," above.

Mature Minor

No specific statute found. But see "Age of Consent," above.

*Louisiana Revised Statutes (1984).

Pregnant Minor, R.S. 40:1299.53

A pregnant minor may consent to medical treatment in connection with the pregnancy.

Minor Parent, R.S. 40:1299.53

A minor parent may consent to care for child, and, although not specifically covered by the statute, may consent for self as well.

Emergency, R.S. 40:1299.54

A physician may provide treatment if it is reasonably necessary, the person authorized to consent is not readily available, and any delay in treatment could reasonably be expected to jeopardize the life or health of the minor or could reasonably result in disfigurement or impaired faculties. Also, case 1 in the text (page 51) is from Louisiana.

Abortion, R.S. 40:1299.35.5

A minor must be eighteen or emancipated judicially or by marriage to consent to an abortion. The minor under eighteen can have the parental consent requirement waived by petitioning the court with juvenile jurisdiction in the parish where she lives or where the abortion is to be performed. The requirement must be waived if the minor is sufficiently mature and well-informed to make the decision or if a waiver is in the best interests of an immature minor.

Contraception

No specific statute found. Please read text for discussion of legal principles.

Sterilization

No specific statute found. Please read text for discussion of legal principles.

Sexually Transmitted Diseases, R.S. 40:1065.1

Any minor may consent to treatment for sexually transmitted diseases. The provider may, but is not required to, notify the parents.

Substance Abuse, R.S. 40:1096

No specific alcohol statute found. But see "Age of Consent," above.

Any minor "who is or believes himself to be addicted to a narcotic or other drug" may be treated. Notification of parents is allowed but not required. This notification provision may violate federal law. (See "Drug and Alcohol Records—Special Privacy Regulations'' in chapter 3.) Addiction is defined to include psychological habituation as well as physical dependence.

Mental Health, Inpatient, R.S. 28:57(B)

Minors sixteen and over may consent to inpatient care. Also, see ''Age of Consent,'' above.

Mental Health, Outpatient

No specific statute found. Please read text for discussion of legal principles. Also, see ''Age of Consent,'' above.

Blood Donation, R.S. 40:1097

Seventeen-year-olds may donate blood but may not receive compensation.

MAINE*

Age of Consent, T.1, §72 (11–A)

The general age of majority is eighteen.

Minor with Other Adult

No specific statute found. Please read text for discussion of legal principles.

Emancipated Minor, T.15, §3506–A

Any juvenile who is sixteen or older, and whose parents refuse to permit the juvenile to live away from home, may request counsel to petition for emancipation. Also, please read text for discussion of legal principles of emancipation.

Mature Minor

No specific statute found. Please read text for discussion of legal principles.

Pregnant Minor

No specific statute found. Please read text for discussion of legal principles.

*Maine Revised Statutes Annotated (1984).

Minor Parent

No specific statute found. Please read text for discussion of legal principles.

Emergency

No specific statute found. Please read text for discussion of legal principles. See also Attorney General Reports, 1959–60, at page 53, where emergency care is recognized as an exception to general consent requirements.

Abortion, T. 22, §1597

Any minor may consent to an abortion. The statute would permit notification of parents for unemancipated minors under seventeen. The notification statute has been preliminarily enjoined by the courts. *Women's Comm. Health Center* v. *Cohen*, 477 F. Supp. 542 (D. Me. 1979).

Contraception, T. 22, §1908

The consent of the parents is required unless the minor is married, or a parent, or would suffer probable health hazards if the services are not provided. This statute is unconstitutional to the extent that mature or emancipated minors may not obtain contraceptives without parental consent. Please see text for discussion of legal principles.

Sterilization, T. 34–B, §7004 (2) (A)

The age of consent is eighteen for unemancipated or unmarried minors. Please read text for discussion of legal principles.

Sexually Transmitted Diseases, T. 32, §§2595, 3292; T. 22, §1823

Any minor may consent to treatment for sexually transmitted diseases. Notification is permitted but not required except parents shall be notified and consent obtained if hospitalization is required and continues beyond sixteen hours.

Substance Abuse, T. 32, §§2595, 3292, 6221; T. 22, §1823

Any minor may consent to care for alcohol or drug abuse. Notification is permitted but not required except the parents shall be notified and consent obtained if hospitalization is required and continues beyond sixteen hours. This notification provision may violate federal law. See "Drug and Alcohol Records—Special Privacy Regulations" in chapter 3.

Mental Health, Inpatient, T. 34–B, §3831

Persons must be eighteen to consent to admission.

Mental Health, Outpatient

No specific statute found. Please read text for discussion of legal principles.

Blood Donation

No specific statute found. Please read text for discussion of legal principles.

MARYLAND*

Age of Consent, Art. 1, §24

The general age of majority is eighteen.

Minor with Other Adult

No specific statute found. Please read text for discussion of legal principles.

Emancipated Minor

No specific statute found. Please read text for discussion of legal principles.

Mature Minor

No specific statute found. Please read text for discussion of legal principles.

Pregnant Minor, Health—General, §20–102(c) (4), (e)

A minor may consent to pregnancy-related care. The physician may notify the parent of the minor. This notification provision is of questionable constitutionality.

Minor Parent, Health—General, §20–102(a)

A minor parent may consent for self and child. Parental notification is permitted but not required.

*Annotated Code of Maryland (1984).

Emergency, Health—General, §20–102(b)

"A minor has the same capacity as an adult to consent to medical treatment if, in the judgment of the attending physician, the life or health of the minor would be affected adversely by delaying treatment to obtain consent of another individual." Notification of parents is permitted but not required.

Abortion, Health—General, §20–103

Any minor may consent to an abortion. The statute requires notification of the parent prior to the abortion unless: (1) the minor does not live with the parents; (2) reasonable efforts at notification were unsuccessful; or (3) notice may lead to physical or emotional abuse of the minor.

The notification provision is probably unconstitutional as applied to mature and emancipated minors. In addition, there is a substantial question whether the statute as applied to immature minors is constitutional because it does not provide an alternate procedure for a determination of whether notification is in the best interests of the minor. Please read text for discussion of legal principles.

Contraception, Health—General, §20–102(c) (5), (e)

Any minor may consent to contraceptive care. Parental notification is permitted, a provision which may be unconstitutional as applied to mature and emancipated minors. Please read text for discussion of constitutional issues.

Sterilization, Health—General, §20–102(c) (5)

Minors may not consent to sterilization.

Sexually Transmitted Diseases, Health—General, §20–102(c) (3), (e)

Any minor may consent to treatment for sexually transmitted diseases. Notification of parents is permitted but not required.

Substance Abuse, Health—General, §20–102(c) (1), (2), (e)

Any minor may consent to drug or alcohol abuse treatment. The provider may, but is not required to, notify the parents. This notification provision may violate federal law. See "Drug and Alcohol Records—Special Privacy Regulations" in chapter 3.

Mental Health, Inpatient, Health—General, §20–104

Minors sixteen and over may consent to admission. Notification of parents is permitted but not required.

Mental Health, Outpatient, Health—General, §20–104

Minors sixteen and over may consent to admission. Notification of parents is permitted but not required.

Blood Donation, Health—General, §20–101

Seventeen-year-olds may donate to voluntary and noncompensatory programs approved by the American Association of Blood Banks or the American Red Cross.

MASSACHUSETTS*

Age of Consent, C.231, §85P

The general age of majority is eighteen.

Minor with Other Adult

No specific statute found. Please read text for discussion of legal principles.

Emancipated Minor, C. 112, §12F

"Any minor may give consent to his medical or dental care . . . if . . . he is living separate and apart from his parent . . . and is managing his own financial affairs."

The health professional may not notify the parents of treatment unless there is a reasonable belief that the life or limb of the minor is endangered. The statute also allows minors who are married, widowed, or divorced, or who are members of the armed forces, to consent to care.

Mature Minor

No specific statute found. Please read text for discussion of legal principles.

Pregnant Minor, C.112, §12F

A pregnant minor may consent to health care. A physician may not notify the parents of treatment unless he or she believes the life or limb of the minor is endangered.

*Annotated Laws of Massachusetts (1985).

Minor Parent, C.112, §12F

A minor parent may consent to care for self and child. A physician may not notify the parents of treatment unless he or she believes the life or limb of the minor is endangered.

Emergency, C.112, §12F

A physician may treat a minor "when delay in treatment [to obtain consent] will endanger the life, limb, or mental well-being of the patient." The records may not be released without the permission of the minor unless the minor's condition is so threatened that life or limb is endangered.

Abortion, C.112, §12S

Unmarried persons must be eighteen to consent to an abortion. A minor who wishes to have the requirement of parental consent waived may petition a judge of the superior court department of the trial court, who must grant the petition if the minor is mature enough to give informed consent to the abortion, or, if she is not mature enough, the abortion would be in her best interests. See *Bellotti* v. *Baird*, 443 U.S. 622 (1979).

Contraception

No specific statute found. Please read text for discussion of legal principles.

Sterilization, C.112, §12F

Minors may not consent to sterilization.

Sexually Transmitted Diseases, C.112, §12F

Any minor may consent to treatment for sexually transmitted diseases. Parental notification may not occur unless the condition of the minor is so serious that life or limb is endangered.

Substance Abuse, C.112, §12E

Minors twelve and over found to be drug-dependent by two or more physicians may give consent to hospital and medical care. This does not apply to methadone maintenance. See also "Mental Health" below.

Mental Health, Inpatient, C.123, §10(a)

A minor may consent to voluntary admission at sixteen.

Mental Health, Outpatient, C.123, §10(b)

A minor may consent to outpatient care at sixteen.

Blood Donation, C.111, §184C

A person must be eighteen to consent to donating blood.

MICHIGAN*

Age of Consent, §722.52, §722.1

The general age of majority is eighteen.

Minor with Other Adult

No specific statute found. Please read text for discussion of legal principles. Note that case 2 in text (page 23), *Bakker* v. *Welsh*, 144 Mich. 632 (1906), is from Michigan.

Emancipated Minor, §722.4

Emancipation occurs during the time that the minor is on active duty with the armed forces, or is validly married, or when the minor is declared to be emancipated by a court of competent jurisdiction. Emancipation also can occur by parents whose conduct clearly indicates intent to release parental rights, or by written agreement of the parent and child filed with the county clerk.

Mature Minor

No specific statute found. Please read text for discussion of legal principles. See also *Bakker* v. *Welsh*, 144 Mich. 632 (1906).

Pregnant Minor

No specific statute found. Please read text for discussion of legal principles.

Minor Parent

No specific statute found. Please read text for discussion of legal principles.

*Michigan Compiled Laws Annotated (1985).

Emergency

No specific statute found. Please read text for discussion of legal principles. See also *Luka* v. *Lowrie*, 136 N.W. 1106 (1912), a leading case on emergency treatment of minors, detailed as case 4 in the text (page 52), which clearly gives physicians the authority to treat minors without parental consent in emergencies.

Abortion

No specific statute found. Please read text for discussion of legal principles. Also, see *Abortion Coalition of Michigan, Inc.* v. *Michigan Dept. of Public Health*, 426 F. Supp. 471 (1977): The state may not impose on an emancipated minor a blanket provision requiring parental consent as a prerequisite to a first-trimester abortion.

Contraception

No specific statute found. Please read text for discussion of legal principles.

Sterilization

No specific statute found. Please read text for discussion of legal principles.

Sexually Transmitted Diseases, §333.5257

Minors may consent to treatment for sexually transmitted diseases. For medical reasons, the provider may, but is not obligated to, notify parents.

Substance Abuse, §333.6121

A minor who is or professes to be suffering from substance abuse may consent to related medical or surgical care, treatment, or services. Notification of parents is permitted for medical reasons, but is not required. To the extent that notification is permitted, it may be in violation of federal law. See "Drug and Alcohol Records—Special Privacy Regulations" in chapter 3.

Mental Health, Inpatient, §330.1411, §330.1415

A person must be eighteen to consent to admission to a facility.

Mental Health, Outpatient

No specific statute found. Please read text for discussion of legal principles.

Blood Donation, §722.41

Seventeen-year-olds may donate blood if the donation is voluntary and no compensation is received.

MINNESOTA*

Age of Consent, §645.45

The general age of majority is eighteen.

Minor with Other Adult

No specific statute found. Please read text for discussion of legal principles.

Emancipated Minor, §144.341, §144.346

"[A]ny minor who is living separate and apart from his parents . . . whether with or without [their] consent . . . and regardless of the duration of such separate residence, and who is managing his own financial affairs, regardless of the source or extent of his income, may give effective consent to dental, mental and other health services." Notification of parents is allowed where failure to do so would seriously jeopardize the health of the minor.

Mature Minor

No specific statute found. Please read text for discussion of legal principles.

Pregnant Minor, §144.343(1), §144.346

A pregnant minor may consent to treatment for pregnancy. Notification of the parent is allowed where failure to do so would seriously jeopardize the health of the minor.

Minor Parent, §144.342, §144.346

A minor parent may consent to care for self and child. Notification of parents is allowed where failure to do so would seriously jeopardize the health of the minor.

*Minnesota Statutes Annotated (1985).

Emergency, §144.344, §144.346

A health care professional may treat a minor without parental consent "when, in the professional's judgment, the risk to the minor's life or health is of such a nature that treatment should be given without delay and the requirement of consent would result in delay or denial of treatment." Notification of the parents is allowed where failure to do so would seriously jeopardize the health of the minor.

Abortion, §144.343

Minors may consent to abortion. Notification of parents of unemancipated minors is required at least forty-eight hours prior to abortion unless (1) there is insufficient time to provide notice; or (2) the minor declares that she is the victim of sexual abuse, neglect, or physical abuse. Notice of such declaration must be made to the proper authorities.

If the notification procedure were ever enjoined by a court, then the statute would allow the minor who did not wish to have her parents notified to petition to a court for a waiver of that requirement. The court would have to grant the waiver if the minor was mature, or if not mature, if the waiver would be in her best interests.

By order effective August 31, 1981, the Minnesota Supreme Court set forth a procedure for waiver of notification of an abortion to the parents of a minor.

Contraception

No specific statute found. Please read text for discussion of legal principles.

Sterilization

No specific statute found. However, state family planning centers must notify a minor's parents when advising sterilization. Please read text for discussion of legal principles.

Sexually Transmitted Diseases, §144.343(1), §144.346

Minors may consent to treatment for sexually transmitted diseases. Parents may be notified when, in the judgment of the professional, failure to do so would seriously jeopardize the health of the minor.

Substance Abuse, §144.343(1), §144.346

Minors may consent to the diagnosis and treatment of alcohol and substance abuse. Parents may be notified when, in the professional's judgment, failure to do so would seriously jeopardize the minor's health. This provision, to the extent that it permits notification, may be in conflict with federal law. See "Drug and Alcohol Records—Special Privacy Regulations" in chapter 3.

Mental Health, Inpatient, §253B.04(1)

Minors sixteen and over may consent to admission.

Mental Health, Outpatient

Emancipated minors, minor parents, and pregnant minors may consent to outpatient care (see statute citations above). For all others, no specific statute found. Please read text for discussion of legal principles.

Blood Donation, §145.41

Seventeen-year-olds may donate blood to voluntary and noncompensatory programs.

MISSISSIPPI*

Age of Consent, §41–41–3(a)

The general age of consent to health care is eighteen.

Minor with Other Adult, §41–41–3

Any adult may consent to medical and surgical treatment for a minor brother or sister. During the absence of a parent, any maternal grandparent, and, if the father is so authorized and the minor is of legitimate birth, any paternal grandparent, may consent for medical or surgical treatment for a minor grandchild. Also, any person standing *in loco parentis*, whether formally serving or not, may consent to medical and surgical treatment of a minor in his or her care. Last, any guardian, conservator, or custodian may consent to medical and surgical care for a ward.

Emancipated Minor, §41–41–3(g)

Emancipated minors may consent to health care.

Mature Minor, §41–41–3(h)

"Any unemancipated minor of sufficient intelligence to understand and

*Mississippi Code, 1972, Annotated (1984).

appreciate the consequences of the proposed surgical or medical treatment or procedures" may consent to care.

Pregnant Minor, §41–41–3(i)

A pregnant minor may consent to care.

Minor Parent, §41–41–3(b)

A minor parent may consent to care for self and child. Note that the father of an illegitimate child may not consent to health care for the child solely on the basis of fatherhood.

Emergency, §41–41–7

A physician may treat a minor when "in competent medical judgment, the proposed surgical or medical treatment or procedures are immediately or imminently necessary and any delay occasioned by an attempt to obtain a consent would reasonably jeopardize the life, health or limb of the person affected, or would reasonably result in disfigurement or impairment of faculties." The statute also permits treatment if there has been a protest or refusal of treatment by a parent followed by a subsequent material or morbid change in the minor's condition and the parent is not immediately available to consent to treatment required by the change in condition.

Abortion

No specific statute found. Please read text for discussion of legal principles.

Contraception, §41–42–7

Contraceptives may be furnished to minors who are parents or married, who have parental consent, or who have been referred by another physician, a clergyman, family planning clinic, school, or state agency. This statute is unconstitutional to the extent that it prevents mature or emancipated minors from obtaining contraceptives without parental consent. Please read text for discussion of legal principles.

Sterilization

No specific statute found. Please read text for discussion of legal principles.

Sexually Transmitted Diseases, §41–41–13

Minors may consent to treatment for sexually transmitted diseases.

Substance Abuse, §41–41–14

Minors fifteen or older may be treated for mental or emotional problems caused by or related to drugs or alcohol. The provider may, but is not required to, notify the parent. This notification provision may conflict with federal laws. See "Drug and Alcohol Records—Special Privacy Regulations" in chapter 3.

Mental Health, Inpatient, §41–21–103(1)

A person must be eighteen or married to consent to admission to a facility.

Mental Health, Outpatient

No specific statute found. Please read text for discussion of legal principles. See also "Substance Abuse," above.

Blood Donation, §41–41–15

Seventeen-year-olds may donate, with or without remuneration, to a licensed hospital, blood bank, community blood program, or other lawful program.

MISSOURI*

Age of Consent, §431.061(1)

The general age of consent to medical treatment is eighteen.

Minor with Other Adult, §431.061(5)–(9)

During the absence of a parent, any adult may consent to medical and surgical treatment of a minor brother or sister. During the absence of a parent, any grandparent may consent to medical and surgical treatment for a minor grandchild. Any adult *in loco parentis*, whether formally or not, may consent to emergency medical care for a minor charge. Last, any guardian may give consent to medical and surgical treatment for a ward.

Emancipated Minor

No specific statute found. Please read text for discussion of legal principles.

*Vernon's Annotated Missouri Statutes (1985).

Mature Minor

No specific statute found. Please read text for discussion of legal principles.

Pregnant Minor, §431.061(4) (a), §431.062

A pregnant minor may consent to care. Physicians may, but are not required to, notify parents of the fact of the minor's pregnancy. This provision is of questionable constitutionality. Note that a physician may *not* notify parents if the pregnancy test is negative.

Minor Parent, §431.061, §431.065

A minor parent may consent for self and child.

Emergency, §431.063

A minor may be treated when "in competent medical judgment, the proposed surgical or medical treatment or procedures are immediately or imminently necessary and any delay occasioned by an attempt to obtain consent would reasonably jeopardize the life, health or limb of the person affected, or would reasonably result in disfigurement or impairment of faculties." The statute also permits treatment if there has been a protest or refusal of treatment by a parent followed by a subsequent material or morbid change in the minor's condition and the parent is not immediately available to consent to treatment required by the change in condition.

Abortion, §188.028

A person must be eighteen or emancipated to consent to an abortion. Minors who wish the parental consent requirement waived may petition the juvenile court, which must grant the petition if the minor is mature enough to make the decision, or if the minor is not mature enough, the abortion would be in her best interests. Because, however, the statute requires that the parents be notified of the court procedure, the statute was declared unconstitutional. *Planned Parenthood* v. *Ashcroft*, 462 U.S. 476 (1983).

Contraception

No specific statute found. Please read text for discussion of legal principles.

Sterilization

No specific statute found. Please read text for discussion of legal principles.

Sexually Transmitted Diseases, §431.061(4) (b), §431.062

Minors may consent to treatment for sexually transmitted diseases. The professional may, but is not required to, notify the parents, but notification may *not* occur if the minor is found not to be suffering from a sexually transmitted disease.

Substance Abuse, §431.06(4) (c), §431.062

No specific statute found for alcohol abuse. Please read text for discussion of legal principles.

Minors may consent to treatment for drug or substance abuse. The parents may, but are not required to, be notified. This notification provision may violate federal law. See "Drug and Alcohol Records—Special Privacy Regulation" in chapter 3. No disclosure may occur if a minor is found *not* to be suffering from drug or substance abuse.

Mental Health, Inpatient, §632.110

A person must be eighteen to consent to admission to a facility.

Mental Health, Outpatient, §632.110

A person must be eighteen to consent to outpatient treatment.

Blood Donation, §431.068

Seventeen-year-olds may donate blood but may not receive compensation without parental consent.

MONTANA*

Age of Consent, §41–1–101

The general age of majority is eighteen.

Minor with Other Adult

No specific statute found. Please read text for a discussion of legal principles.

Emancipated Minor, §41–1–402(1) (a) and (b), §41–1–403

Minors who have graduated from high school, or who are emancipated, or live separate and apart from their parents for whatever reason and are self-supporting by whatever means, may consent to medical treatment.

*Montana Code Annotated (1984).

The health professional may notify such a minor's parents of the treatment when (1) severe complications are anticipated or major surgery or prolonged hospitalization is needed; or (2) failure to do so would seriously jeopardize the minor, younger siblings, or the public; or (3) notification would benefit the minor's physical and mental health and family harmony, or the hospital desires a third-party commitment to pay for services rendered or to be rendered. Disclosure, however, is not required.

Mature Minor

No specific statute found. Please read text for a discussion of legal principles.

Pregnant Minor, §41–1–402(1) (c), §41–1–403

A pregnant minor may consent to treatment. Notification is permitted as set forth in "Emancipated Minor," above. Note that such notification may be constitutionally suspect to the extent that it permits the notification of the parents of mature or emancipated minors. Note that the parents may *not* be notified if the minor is found not to be pregnant.

Minor Parent, §41–1–402 (2), §41–1–403

A minor parent may consent to care for self and child. Notification of the minor's parent is permitted as set forth in "Emancipated Minor," above.

Emergency, §41–1–405

"Any health professional may render or attempt to render emergency service or first aid, medical, surgical, dental or psychiatric treatment, without compensation, to any injured person or any person regardless of age who is in need of immediate health care when, in good faith, the professional believes that the giving of aid is the only alternative to probable death or serious physical or mental damage."

Also: "Any health professional may render nonemergency services to minors for conditions which will endanger the health or life of the minor if services would be delayed by obtaining consent from spouse, parent, parents, or legal guardian."

See also §41–1–402(1) (d), which allows a hospital, public clinic, or physician to provide emergency care, without which the minor's health will be jeopardized, without parental consent. While §41–1–405 is silent regarding parental notification after treatment is provided, §41–1–402 requires such notification.

Abortion, §50–20–107

Minors may consent to abortions. Written notice must be given to the parents of the minor if she is under eighteen years of age and unmarried.

The notification provision is most likely unconstitutional as applied to mature or emancipated minors. In addition, there are substantial questions whether the statute is constitutional as applied to immature minors because it does not provide an alternate procedure for a determination of whether notification is in the best interests of an immature minor. See *Doe* v. *Deschamps*, 461 F. Supp. 682 (D. Mont. 1976). Please read text for discussion of legal principles.

Contraception

No specific statute found. Please read text for discussion of legal principles.

Sterilization, §41–1–405(4)

Minors may not consent to sterilizations.

Sexually Transmitted Diseases, §41–1–402(1)(c), §41–1–403

Minors may consent to treatment for sexually transmitted diseases. Notification is permitted as set forth in "Emancipated Minor," above. But notification is *not* allowed if the minor is found not to be suffering from a venereal disease.

Substance Abuse, §41–1–402(1)(c), §41–1–403

Minors who profess or are found to be afflicted with alcohol or drug abuse problems may be treated. Notification of parents is permitted as set forth in "Emancipated Minor," above. But notification is *not* allowed if the minor is found not to be suffering from drug or alcohol abuse. To the extent that notification is permitted, it may violate federal law. See "Drug and Alcohol Records—Special Privacy Regulations" in chapter 3.

Mental Health, Inpatient, §53–21–112

Minors sixteen and over may consent to admission to state facilities. Also, if, in any application for voluntary admission for any period of time to a mental health facility, a minor fails to join in the consent of his parents or guardian to the voluntary admission, then the application for admission shall be treated as a petition for involuntary commitment.

Mental Health, Outpatient, §53–21–112

Minors sixteen and over may consent to outpatient treatment. Also, §41–1–406 permits minors to consent to psychiatric or psychological counseling when the need for such counseling is urgent in the opinion of the physician or psychologist involved, and the consent of a parent cannot be obtained within a reasonable time to offset the danger to life or safety.

Blood Donation

No specific statute found. Please read text for a discussion of legal principles.

NEBRASKA*

Age of Consent, §38–101

The general age of majority is nineteen. Also, married minors are considered adults.

Minor with Other Adult

No specific statute found. Please read text for discussion of legal principles.

Emancipated Minor

No specific statute found. Pleaes read text for discussion of legal principles.

Mature Minor

No specific statute found. Please read text for discussion of legal principles.

Pregnant Minor

No specific statute found. Please read text for discussion of legal principles.

Minor Parent

No specific statute found. Please read text for discussion of legal principles.

Emergency, §71–5512

"[E]mergency medical, surgical, hospital or health services [may be provided] to any individual, regardless of age" when the patient is unable to consent to treatment and there is no other person reasonably available to consent. This statute specifically relieves enumerated professionals from civil liability solely for failure to obtain parental consent before providing a minor with emergency treatment.

*Revised Statutes of Nebraska (1984).

Abortion, §28–347

Minors may consent to abortions. Notice must be given to parents of a minor at least twenty-four hours before the abortion. A minor who does not wish notification to occur may petition a district court for a waiver, which must be granted if the minor is mature enough to make the decision or notification would not be in the minor's best interests. See *Orr* v. *Knowles*, 337 N.W.2d 699 (1983).

Contraception

No specific statute found. Please read text for discussion of legal principles.

Sterilization

No specific statute found. Please read text for discussion of legal principles.

Sexually Transmitted Diseases, §71–1121

Minors may consent to treatment for sexually transmitted diseases. Parents are liable for expenses for treatment of children in their custody. Also, reasonable care must be taken to "elicit from any such person who is under twenty years of age any history of sensitivity or previous adverse reaction to medication."

Substance Abuse, §71–5041

Minors may be treated for alcohol and drug abuse. The health care provider shall attempt to involve the family, but failure to obtain parental consent before treating a minor who understands the treatment shall not result in liability.

Mental Health, Inpatient

No specific statute found. Please read text for discussion of legal principles.

Mental Health, Outpatient

No specific statute found. Please read text for discussion of legal principles.

Blood Donation, §71–4808

Seventeen-year-olds may donate blood but may not receive compensation without parental consent.

NEVADA*

Age of Consent, §129.010

The general age of majority is eighteen.

Minor with Other Adult, §129.040

When a minor's parents cannot be located after reasonable efforts, any person standing *in loco parentis* to the minor may give consent to emergency treatment.

Emancipated Minor, §129.030(1) (a)

"A minor may give consent for . . . [health care services] . . . for himself . . . if he is living apart from his parents . . . with or without . . . [their] consent . . . and has so lived for a period of at least 4 months."

Mature Minor, §129.030(2)

The consent of the parent is not necessary to treat a minor "who understands the nature and purpose of the proposed examination or treatment and its probable outcome and voluntarily requests it." This statute does not cover sterilization.

Pregnant Minor

No specific statute found. Please read text for a discussion of legal principles. See also "Mature Minor," above.

Minor Parent, §129.030(1) (c)

A minor who has borne a child or is a mother may consent to treatment for self and child.

Emergency, §129.030(1) (d), (3)

Any minor may consent to treatment if, in the physician's judgment, the minor will suffer a serious health hazard if health services are not provided.

"A person who treats a minor [for emergency care] shall, before initiating treatment, make prudent and reasonable efforts to obtain his consent to communicate with his parent, parents or legal guardian, and shall make a note of such efforts in the record of his care. If the person believes that such efforts would jeopardize treatment necessary to the minor's life or necessary to avoid a serious and immediate threat to the minor's health, the person may omit such efforts and note the reasons for the omission in the record."

*Nevada Revised Statutes (1983).

Abortion, §442.255

Minors may consent to abortions. Notification to parents of unmarried and unemancipated minors is required at least twenty-four hours before the abortion.

The notification provision has been preliminarily enjoined; *Glick* v. *McKay*, 616 F.Supp. 322 (D. Nev. 1985). Please read text for discussion of constitutional principles.

Contraception

No specific statute found. Please read text for a discussion of legal principles. See also "Mature Minor," above.

Sterilization, §129.030(4)

The general medical consent statute states that a minor may not consent to sterilization.

Sexually Transmitted Diseases, §129.060

Minors may consent to treatment for sexually transmitted diseases. See also §441.175.

Substance Abuse, §129.050

No specific statute found for alcohol abuse. Please read text for a discussion of legal principles and see "Mature Minor," above.

Minors under the influence or suspected of being under the influence of a controlled substance or dangerous or hallucinogenic drug may be treated. The health care provider shall make every reasonable effort to report the fact of treatment to the parents within a reasonable time thereafter. The notification provision may conflict with federal law. See "Drug and Alcohol Records—Special Privacy Regulations" in chapter 3.

Mental Health, Inpatient, §433A.140

Any person may apply for admission to public or private mental health facilities.

Mental Health, Outpatient

No specific statute found. Please read text for a discussion of legal principles. Also, see "Mature Minor," above.

Blood Donation, §460.040

Any person who is seventeen or older may donate blood without parental consent.

NEW HAMPSHIRE*

Age of Consent, §21–B:1 (1983)

The general age of majority is eighteen.

Minor with Other Adult

No specific statute found. Please read text for a discussion of legal principles.

Emancipated Minor

No specific statute found. Please read text for a discussion of legal principles. See "Mature Minor," below.

Mature Minor, §318–B: 12–a (1984)

A minor may consent to medical treatment "provided that such minor is of sufficient maturity to understand the nature of such treatment and the consequences thereof."

Pregnant Minor

No specific statute found. Please read text for a discussion of legal principles and see "Mature Minor," above.

Minor Parent

No specific statute found. Please read text for a discussion of legal principles and see "Mature Minor," above.

Emergency

No statute on this point was found. But see RS 627:6 (VII) (1983), which releases a physician or persons acting under a physician's direction from criminal liability for treating a minor under emergency circumstances. See also 507:8–d (1983), which relieves a person from civil liability for acts which were taken pursuant to the provision of emergency care. The two statutes read together have the effect of releasing the health service provider of any civil or criminal liability for providing emergency treatment without parental consent.

Abortion

No specific statute found. Please read text for a discussion of legal principles. See also "Mature Minor," above.

*New Hampshire Revised Statutes (date of latest supplement appears after each statute cited).

Contraception

No specific statute found. Please read text for a discussion of legal principles. See also "Mature Minor," above.

Sterilization, §460:21–a (1983)

Minors may not consent to sterilizations.

Sexually Transmitted Diseases, §141:11–a (1983)

Minors fourteen and over may consent to treatment for sexually transmitted diseases.

Substance Abuse, §318–B:12–a (1984)

No specific statute found. Please read text for a discussion of legal principles. See also "Mature Minor," above.

Minors twelve and over may be treated for drug dependency or any problem related to the use of drugs.

Mental Health, Inpatient, §135–B:11 (1983)

Anyone who is eighteen may consent to admission to a mental health facility. The Director of Mental Health is required by statute to establish eligibility requirements for minors applying for admission and procedures for parental notification.

Mental Health, Outpatient

No specific statute found. Please read text for a discussion of legal principles. See also "Mature Minor," above.

Blood Donation, §571–C:1 (1983)

Minors seventeen and over or married may donate blood to any voluntary and noncompensatory program.

NEW JERSEY*

Age of Consent, §9:17B–1(a)

The general age of majority is eighteen.

Minor with Other Adult

No specific statute found. Please read text for a discussion of legal principles.

*New Jersey Statutes Annotated (1984).

Emancipated Minor

No specific statute found. Please read text for a discussion of legal principles.

Mature Minor

No specific statute found. Please read text for a discussion of legal principles.

Pregnant Minor, §9:17A–1, §9:17A–5

A pregnant minor may consent to treatment. The statute permits notification of the parents of the minor and is of questionable constitutionality.

Minor Parent, §9:17A–1, §9:17A–5

A minor may consent for self and child. The statute would permit notification of the minor's parents.

Emergency

No specific statute found. Please read text for a discussion of legal principles.

Abortion

No specific statute found. Please read text for discussion of legal principles.

Contraception

No specific statute found. Please read text for discussion of legal principles.

Sterilization

No specific statute found. Please read text for a discussion of legal principles.

Sexually Transmitted Diseases, §9:17A–4, §9:17A–5

Minors may consent to treatment for sexually transmitted diseases. Parents of the minor may be notified of the treatment but are not required to be.

Substance Abuse, §9:17A–4, §9:17A–5

No specific statute found regarding alcohol abuse. Please read text for a discussion of legal principles.

A minor who believes he is suffering from drug abuse or who is drug-dependent may be treated. The parents may be notified, but are not required to be. This notification provision may violate federal law. See "Drug and Alcohol Records—Special Privacy Regulations" in chapter 3.

Mental Health, Inpatient, §30:4–46

A person must be eighteen to sign into a facility. The New Jersey courts have ruled that minors who have been admitted by their parents to private or public hospitals have the right to sign themselves out on seventy-two hours' notice without parental consent.

Mental Health, Outpatient

No specific statute found. Please read text for a discussion of legal principles.

Blood Donation, §9:17A–6

A person must be eighteen to donate blood.

NEW MEXICO*

Age of Consent, §28–6–1

The general age of majority is eighteen.

Minor with Other Adult

No specific statute found. Please read text for a discussion of legal principles.

Emancipated Minor, §28–6–2 through §28–6–8; §24–10–1

Emancipated minors (meaning those who have entered into valid marriages, are on active duty in the armed forces, or have been declared emancipated by the children's court) may consent to medical, dental, or psychiatric care. Note that the definition of emancipation set out in the statute does not include minors who have not been formally declared emancipated but who live apart from their parents, are self-supporting, and managing their own financial affairs. These minors, as well, may consent to medical treatment. Please see text for discussion of legal principles.

*New Mexico Statutes Annotated (1984).

Mature Minor

No specific statute found. Please read text for a discussion of legal principles.

Pregnant Minor, §24–1–13

"Any person, regardless of age, has the capacity to consent to an examination and diagnosis by a licensed physician for pregnancy."

Minor Parent

No specific statute found. Please read text for a discussion of legal principles.

Emergency, §24–10–2

A minor may be treated when "in need of immediate hospitalization, medical attention or surgery and the parents of the minor cannot be located for the purpose of consenting thereto, after reasonable efforts have been made under the circumstances."

Abortion, §30–5–1(c)

This statute has been declared unconstitutional in part. Please read text for general discussion of constitutional principles.

Contraception, §24–8–3, §24–8–5

Minors may consent to contraceptive care.

Sterilization

No specific statute found. Please read text for a discussion of legal principles.

Sexually Transmitted Diseases, §24–1–9

Minors may consent to treatment for sexually transmitted diseases.

Substance Abuse, §26–2–14

No specific statute found for alcohol abuse. Please read text for a discussion of legal principles.

Any minor may be treated for drug abuse and the parents may not be notified.

Mental Health, Inpatient, 43–1–16

Minors twelve and over may voluntarily admit themselves to facilities; however, the parent or guardian must also consent to the admission. The statute also permits minors twelve and over to object to or terminate the admission.

Mental Health, Outpatient

No specific statute found. Please read text for a discussion of legal principles.

Blood Donation

No specific statute found. Please read text for a discussion of legal principles.

NEW YORK*

Age of Consent, Public Health Law, §2504

The general age of consent to health care is eighteen.

Minor with Other Adult

No specific statute found. Please read text for a discussion of legal principles.

Emancipated Minor

No specific statute found. Please read text for a discussion of legal principles. See also Public Health Law, §2504(2), which states that any minor who has been married may consent to health care.

Mature Minor

No specific statute found. Please read text for a discussion of legal principles. Also see *Bach* v. *Long Island Jewish Hospital*, 267 N.Y.S.2d 289 (Sup. Ct. 1966), presented as case 1 in the text (page 44), which is from New York.

Pregnant Minor, Public Health Law, §2504(3)

Any minor who is pregnant may consent to medical, dental, health, and hospital services relating to prenatal care.

*McKinney's Consolidated Laws of New York Annotated (1984).

Minor Parent, Public Health Law, §2504(2)

Any minor who has borne a child may consent to care for self and child.

Emergency, Public Health Law, §2504(4)

"[W]hen, in the physician's judgment an emergency exists and the person is in immediate need of medical attention and an attempt to secure consent would result in delay of treatment which would increase the risk to the person's life or health," treatment may proceed.

Abortion

No specific statute found. Please read text for a discussion of legal principles.

Contraception

No specific statute found. Please read text for a discussion of legal principles. See *Carey* v. *Population Services,* 431 U.S. 678 (1977), in which the Supreme Court declared unconstitutional a statute which prohibited the distribution of contraceptives to minors under sixteen.

Sterilization

No specific statute found. Please read text for discussion of legal principles.

Sexually Transmitted Diseases, Public Health Law, §2305(2)

Minors may consent to treatment for sexually transmitted diseases.

Substance Abuse, Mental Hygiene Law, §21.11, §23.01(a) (2)

This statute allows treatment for alcohol abuse and alcoholism without parental consent if the requirement of consent would be detrimental to treatment, or the parent refuses consent and the physician believes the treatment to be in the best interests of the minor. The minor must be advised of the availability of advocacy services and must sign a consent that the treatment is voluntary and that certain information required was provided.

Mental Health, Inpatient, Mental Hygiene Law, §9.13(a)

Minors may consent to admission at sixteen.

Mental Health, Outpatient, Mental Hygiene Law, §33.21

Minors may consent to indicated outpatient care when the requirement of parental consent would be detrimental to treatment.

Blood Donation, Public Health Law, §3123

Seventeen-year-olds may donate blood to voluntary and noncompensatory programs.

NORTH CAROLINA*

Age of Consent, §48A–2

The general age of majority is eighteen.

Minor with Other Adult

No specific statute found. Please read text for discussion of legal principles.

Emancipated Minor, §90–21.5(b)

"Any minor who is emancipated may consent to any medical treatment, dental and health services for himself or his child."

Mature Minor

No specific statute found. Please read text for discussion of legal principles.

Pregnant Minor, §90–21.5(a) (ii), §90–21.4(b)

Pregnant minors may consent to health care. Notification to parents is allowed when essential to the life or health of the minor.

Minor Parent, §90–21.5(b)

Any minor who is emancipated may consent to any medical treatment, dental and health services for self or child. Note that minors who are parents and live with their parents may also consent to care for self and child. Please read text for discussion of legal principles.

Emergency, §90–21.1

When the parents cannot be contacted with reasonable diligence during which time the minor needs to receive treatment, or when the identity of the child is unknown or when the necessity for treatment is so apparent that an effort to obtain consent would result in a delay which would endanger the life of the minor, or when an effort to obtain consent would result in delay which would seriously worsen the condition of the minor, treatment may proceed.

*General Statutes of North Carolina (1984).

When surgery is contemplated, a second opinion must be obtained when possible. The statute also permits treatment when a parent refuses treatment and the "necessity for immediate treatment is so apparent that the delay required to obtain a court order would endanger the life or seriously worsen the physical condition of the child."

Abortion

No specific statute found. Please read text for discussion of legal principles.

Contraception, §90–21.5(a) (ii), §90–21.4(b)

Minors may consent to contraceptive treatment. Notification to parents is allowed when essential to the life or health of the minor.

Sterilization, §§90–271, 272

Married minors may consent to sterilization. Unmarried minors may not be sterilized without a court order.

Sexually Transmitted Diseases, §90–21.5(a) (i), §90–21.4(b)

Minors may consent to treatment for sexually transmitted diseases. Parental notification is allowed when essential to the life or health of the minor.

Substance Abuse, §90–21.5(a) (iii), §90–21.4(b)

Treatment may be provided to minors for the prevention, diagnosis, and treatment of alcohol abuse and the abuse of controlled substances. Notification of parents is allowed when essential to the life or health of the minor. This notification provision may violate federal law. See "Drug and Alcohol Records—Special Privacy Regulations" in chapter 3.

Mental Health, Inpatient, §90–21.5

Emancipated minors may consent to admission to a facility. Otherwise a person must be eighteen.

Mental Health, Outpatient, §90–21.5(a) (iv)

Minors may consent to medical health services for the prevention, diagnosis, and treatment of emotional disturbance, short of commitment to a mental institution or hospital for confinement or treatment of a mental condition.

Blood Donation, §90–220.11

Seventeen-year-olds may donate blood but may not receive compensation.

NORTH DAKOTA*

Age of Consent, §14–10–01

The general age of majority is eighteen.

Minor with Other Adult

No specific statute found. Please read text for a discussion of legal principles.

Emancipated Minor

No specific statute found. Please read text for a discussion of legal principles.

Mature Minor

No specific statute found. Please read text for a discussion of legal principles.

Pregnant Minor

No specific statute found. Please read text for discussion of legal principles.

Minor Parent

No specific statute found. Please read text for a discussion of legal principles.

Emergency, §14–10–17.1

"Any minor may contract for and receive emergency examination, care, or treatment in a life threatening situation without permission, authority, or consent of parent or guardian."

Abortion, §14–02.1–03, §14–02.1–03.1

A person must be eighteen to consent to an abortion unless emancipated. Other minors may petition a juvenile court in order to waive the parental

*North Dakota Century Code (1983).

consent requirement. The petition will be granted if the minor is mature enough to make the decision or if granting the petition would be in her best interests.

Contraception

No specific statute found. Please read text for discussion of legal principles.

Sterilization

No specific statute found. Please read text for a discussion of legal principles.

Sexually Transmitted Diseases, §14–10–17

Minors fourteen and over may consent to treatment for sexually transmitted diseases.

Substance Abuse, §14–10–17

Minors fourteen and over may be treated for alcoholism or drug abuse.

Mental Health, Inpatient, §25–03.1–04

A person must be eighteen to consent to admission to a facility.

Mental Health, Outpatient

No specific statute found. Please read text for a discussion of legal principles.

Blood Donation

A statute which required that persons be eighteen in order to donate blood was repealed in 1983.

OHIO*

Age of Consent, §3109.01

The general age of majority is eighteen.

Minor with Other Adult

No specific statute found. Please read text for a discussion of legal principles.

*Ohio Revised Code (1984).

Emancipated Minor

No specific statute found. Please read text for a discussion of legal principles.

Mature Minor

No specific statute found. See *Lacey* v. *Laird*, 139 N.E. 2d 25 (1956), presented as case 3 in the text (page 217), which is from Ohio.

Pregnant Minor

No specific statute found. Please read text for a discussion of legal principles.

Minor Parent

No specific statute found. Please read text for a discussion of legal principles.

Emergency

No specific statute found. Please read text for a discussion of legal principles.

Abortion, §2919.12

Persons must be eighteen or married to consent to abortions. This statute has been declared unconstitutional. *Hoe* v. *Brown*, 446 F. Supp. 329 (1976). Please read text for a general discussion of constitutional principles.

Contraception

No specific statute found. Please read text for a discussion of legal principles.

Sterilization

No specific statute found. Please read text for a discussion of legal principles.

Sexually Transmitted Diseases, §3709.241

Minors may consent to treatment for sexually transmitted diseases.

Substance Abuse, §3719.012

No specific statute found for alcohol abuse. Please read text for a discussion of legal principles.

Minors may be treated for any condition which is reasonably believed to be caused by drug abuse.

Mental Health, Inpatient, §5122.02

A person must be eighteen to consent to admission to a facility.

Mental Health, Outpatient

No specific statute found. Please read text for a discussion of legal principles.

Blood Donation, §2108.21

Any person seventeen or older may donate blood.

OKLAHOMA*

Age of Consent, T. 15, §13

The general age of majority is eighteen. See also T. 10, §170.

Minor with Other Adult

No specific statute found. Please read text for a discussion of legal principles.

Emancipated Minor, T. 63, §2602(A) (1), (2); §2604

"Any minor who . . . is emancipated [or] . . . is separated from his parents or legal guardian for whatever reason and is not supported by his parents or legal guardian" may consent to medical care.

The health professional may, but is not required to, notify the parents of treatment. When major surgery, general anesthesia, or a life-threatening procedure is called for, the physician must obtain a concurring opinion except in an emergency in a community where no other surgeon can be contacted within a reasonable time.

Mature Minor

No specific statute found. Please read text for a discussion of legal principles.

Pregnant Minor, T. 63, §2602(A) (3); §2604

Minors may consent to pregnancy care. Physicians may, but are not required to, notify the parents of the care. This notification provision may

*Oklahoma Statutes Annotated (1984).

be of questionable constitutionality. Also, the physician may *not* notify the parent if the pregnancy test is negative. When major surgery, general anesthesia, or a life-threatening procedure is called for, the physician must obtain a concurring opinion except in an emergency in a community where no other surgeon can be contacted within a reasonable time.

Minor Parent, T. 63, §2602(A) (1), (4)

Any parent may consent to care for self and child.

Emergency, T. 63, §2602(A) (7); §2604

A minor may consent to treatment for "conditions which will endanger his health or life" if treatment would be delayed by attempting to obtain parental consent. Reasonable attempts to notify parents of emergency treatment must occur.

Pregnancy prevention is not considered emergency care. Also, when major surgery, general anesthesia, or a life-threatening procedure is called for, the physician must obtain a concurring opinion except in an emergency in a community where no other surgeon can be contacted within a reasonable time.

Abortion

No specific statute found. Please read text for a discussion of legal principles. See T. 63 §1–730 et seq. for general abortion statute.

Contraception

No specific statute found. See 1979 Op. Att'y Gen. No. 79–121, in which the Attorney General stated that parental consent to obtain contraceptive care was not required for a minor who had been married or divorced. Note that a much broader class of minors may consent to contraceptive care. Please read text for a discussion of legal principles.

Sterilization

No specific statute found. Please read text for discussion of legal principles.

Sexually Transmitted Diseases, T. 63, §§2602(A) (3), 2604

Minors may consent to treatment for sexually transmitted diseases. The health professional may, but is not required to, notify the minor's parents. Notification is *not* allowed when the minor is found not to be suffering from a sexually transmitted disease. Finally, the health professional who accepts the responsibility of providing treatment for such diseases also accepts the responsibility to provide some counseling to the minor.

Last, when major surgery, general anesthesia, or a life-threatening procedure is called for, the physician must obtain a concurring opinion except in an emergency in a community where no other surgeon can be contacted within a reasonable time.

Substance Abuse, T. 63, §2602(A) (3); §2604

Minors may consent to treatment for alcohol or drug abuse. Notification is permitted but not required but notification may *not* occur if the minor is determined not to be suffering from substance abuse. The notification provision, to the extent that it permits notification, may be in violation of federal law. See "Drug and Alcohol Records—Special Privacy Regulations" in chapter 3. Last, when major surgery, general anesthesia, or a life-threatening procedure is called for, the physician must obtain a concurring opinion except in an emergency in a community where no other surgeon can be contacted within a reasonable time.

Mental Health, Inpatient, T. 63, §2602

Any minor who is married, has a dependent child, is emancipated, or is separated from his parents for whatever reason and is not supported by his parents may consent to admission.

Mental Health, Outpatient, T. 63, §2602

Any minor who is married, has a dependent child, is emancipated, or is separated from his parents for whatever reason and is not supported by his parents may consent to outpatient treatment.

Blood Donation, T. 63, §2152

Seventeen-year-olds may donate blood with parental permission but not for compensation.

OREGON*

Age of Consent, §109.640, §109.650

Minors fifteen or older may consent to hospital, medical, and surgical care. The physician is allowed to notify the parents of treatment.

Minor with Other Adult

No specific statute found. Please read text for a discussion of legal principles.

*Oregon Revised Statutes (1983).

Emancipated Minor

No specific medical consent statute found, but see "Age of Consent," above. Also, please read text for a discussion of legal principles.

Mature Minor

No specific statute found. Please read text for a discussion of legal principles. See also "Age of Consent," above.

Pregnant Minor

No specific statute found, but see "Age of Consent," above. Also, please read text for a discussion of legal principles.

Minor Parent

No specific statute found, but see "Age of Consent," above. Also, please read text for a discussion of legal principles.

Emergency

No specific statute found. Please read text for a discussion of legal principles. Also, see "Age of Consent," above.

Abortion

No specific statute found. Please read text for a discussion of legal principles. Also, see "Age of Consent," above.

Contraception, §109.640, §109.650

Minors may consent to contraceptive health care at fifteen. This statute is probably unconstitutional to the extent it prevents mature or emancipated minors under fifteen from obtaining contraceptives without parental consent. Please see text for discussion of legal principles. Also, parental notification is not permitted under this statute.

Sterilization, §436.205, §436.225

Minors fifteen and over who can give informed consent may consent to sterilization. But read text for legal principles which may limit this provision.

Sexually Transmitted Diseases, §109.610

Minors may consent to treatment for sexually transmitted diseases.

Substance Abuse

No specific statute found, but see "Age of Consent," above. Also, please read text for a discussion of legal principles.

Mental Health, Inpatient, §426.220

A person must be eighteen to consent to admission to a facility.

Mental Health, Outpatient

No specific statute found. Please read text for a discussion of legal principles. Also, see "Age of Consent," above.

Blood Donation, §109.670

Sixteen-year-olds may donate blood to voluntary and noncompensatory programs approved by the Red Cross or Association of Blood Banks.

PENNSYLVANIA*

Age of Consent, T. 35, §10101

The general age of consent to health care is eighteen. Also, minors who have graduated from high school or who are married may consent to medical, health, or dental services.

Minor with Other Adult

No specific statute found. Please read text for a discussion of legal principles.

Emancipated Minor

No specific statute found. Please read text for a discussion of legal principles. Also, see "Age of Consent," above.

Mature Minor

No specific statute found. Please read text for a discussion of legal principles. Also, see "Age of Consent," above.

Pregnant Minor, T. 35, §§10101, 10103

Pregnant minors may consent to treatment, as may minors who have been pregnant in the past.

*Purdon's Pennsylvania Statutes Annotated (1985).

Minor Parent, T. 35, §10102

A minor parent may consent to care for self and child.

Emergency, T. 35, §10104

A minor may be treated without parental consent "when, in the physician's judgment, an attempt to secure consent would result in delay of treatment which would increase the risk to the minor's life or health."

Abortion, T. 18, §3206

A person must be eighteen to consent to an abortion unless she is emancipated or an emergency exists.

A minor may petition the court of common pleas for a waiver of the parental consent requirement, which must be granted if the minor is mature enough to make the decision, or if the minor is not mature enough to make the decision but the waiver would be in her best interests.

Contraception

No specific statute found. Please read text for a discussion of legal principles. Also, see "Age of Consent," above.

Sterilization

No specific statute found. Please read text for discussion of legal principles.

Sexually Transmitted Diseases, T. 35, §10103

Minors may consent to treatment for sexually transmitted diseases.

Substance Abuse, T. 71, §1690.112

No specific statute found for alcohol abuse. Please read text for a discussion of legal principles. Also, see "Age of Consent."

A minor who suffers from the use of a controlled substance or a harmful substance may consent to treatment. Notification of parents is permitted but not required. This notification provision may violate federal law. See "Drug and Alcohol Records—Special Privacy Regulations" in chapter 3.

Mental Health, Inpatient, T. 50, §§7201, 7204

Minors fourteen and over who substantially understand the nature of the voluntary treatment may consent to admission. Upon acceptance of an application for examination and treatment by a minor fourteen and over but under eighteen, the director of the facility shall promptly notify the minor's parents and shall inform them of the right to be heard upon the filing of an objection.

Mental Health, Outpatient

No specific statute found. Please read text for a discussion of legal principles. Also, see "Age of Consent," above.

Blood Donation, T. 35, §10001

A person must be eighteen to donate blood.

RHODE ISLAND*

Age of Consent, §15–12–1

The general age of majority is eighteen.

Minor with Other Adult

No specific statute found. Please read text for discussion of legal principles.

Emancipated Minor

No specific statute found. Please read text for discussion of legal principles.

Mature Minor

No specific statute found. Please read text for discussion of legal principles.

Pregnant Minor

No specific statute found. Please read text for discussion of legal principles.

Minor Parent, §23–4.6–1

A minor parent may consent to the treatment of his or her child. Also, although not specifically set forth in the statute, a minor parent may consent for self as well.

*General Laws of Rhode Island, 1956, Reenactment of 1979 (1984).

Emergency, §23–4.6–1

"Any person of the age of sixteen or over or married may consent to routine emergency medical or surgical care."

This statute is rather confusing because the words "routine" and "emergency" seem to be mutually exclusive, and no cases were found clarifying this confusion. Also, because the statute speaks in terms of the ability of the minor to consent to care, the informed consent of the minor must be obtained. Last, for minors under sixteen, the legal principles described in the text would be applicable.

Abortion, §23–4.7–6

A person must be eighteen to consent to an abortion unless married or judicially emancipated.

A minor may have the parental consent requirement waived by petitioning the family court, which must grant the petition if the minor is mature enough to make the decision, or if the abortion would be in her best interests.

Contraception

No specific statute found. Please read text for discussion of legal principles.

Sterilization, §11–9–17

A person must be eighteen to consent to sterilization unless the procedure is necessary to preserve a minor's life or health. Also, read text for discussion of legal principles.

Sexually Transmitted Diseases, §23–11–11

Any minor may consent to treatment for sexually transmitted diseases. Notification of parents is not permitted.

Substance Abuse, §40.1–4–9

Any alcoholic minor may consent to treatment. No specific statute was found regarding drug abuse. Please see text for discussion of legal principles.

Mental Health, Inpatient, §40.1–5–6

A person must be eighteen to consent to admission to a facility.

Mental Health, Outpatient

No specific statute found. Please read text for discussion of legal principles.

Blood Donations, §23–4.5–1

A person must be eighteen to donate blood.

SOUTH CAROLINA*

Age of Consent, §20–7–280

Minors sixteen and over may consent to medical care, but not to operations unless essential to the life or health of the minor and unless a consulting physician, if available, agrees. This is not a general age-of-majority statute.

Minor with Other Adult

No specific statute found. Please read text for discussion of legal principles.

Emancipated Minor

No specific statute found. Please read text for discussion of legal principles. Also, see "Age of Consent," above.

Mature Minor

No specific statute found. Please read text for discussion of legal principles. See "Age of Consent," above.

Pregnant Minor, §20–7–300

No specific statute found. Please read text for discussion of legal principles. Also see "Age of Consent," above.

Minor Parents, §20–7–300

Any minor who has borne a child may consent to care for the child, and, although not specifically set forth in the statute, may consent to care for self.

*Code of Law of South Carolina, 1976 (1985).

Emergency, §20–7–290

"Health services of any kind may be rendered to minors . . . without the consent of a parent . . . when, in the judgment of a person authorized by law to render a particular health service, such services are deemed necessary unless such involves an operation which shall be performed only if such is essential to the health or life of such child in the opinion of the performing physician and a consultant physician if one is available."

Abortion, §44–41–30(b)

This statute has been declared unconstitutional. *Floyd* v. *Abrams*, 440 F.Supp. 535 (three-judge court), vacated, 440 U.S. 445, reh. den., 441 U.S. 928 (1979). Please read text for general discussion of constitutional principles.

Contraception

No specific statute found. See "Age of Consent," above. See also 1971–72 Op. Att'y Gen. 213, where the Attorney General stated that minors age sixteen years and older are authorized to procure birth control without the consent of their parents or other persons. Minors younger than sixteen, however, are also constitutionally permitted to procure birth control without parental consent if mature enough to give informed consent. Please read text for discussion of legal principles.

Sterilization

No specific statute found. Please read text for discussion of legal principles.

Sexually Transmitted Diseases

No specific statute found. Please read text for discussion of legal principles. Also, see "Age of Consent," above.

Substance Abuse

No specific statute found. Please read text for discussion of legal principles. Also, see "Age of Consent," above.

Mental Health, Inpatient, §44–17–310

Minors may consent to admission to a facility at sixteen.

Mental Health, Outpatient, §20–7–280

Minors sixteen and over may consent to outpatient treatment.

Blood Donation, §44–43–20

Seventeen-year-olds may consent to blood donation but may not receive compensation without parental consent.

SOUTH DAKOTA*

Age of Consent, §26–1–1

The general age of majority is eighteen.

Minor with Other Adult

No specific statute found. Please read text for discussion of legal principles.

Emancipated Minor

No specific statute found. Please read text for discussion of legal principles.

Mature Minor

No specific statute found. Please read text for discussion of legal principles.

Pregnant Minor

No specific statute found. Please read text for discussion of legal principles.

Minor Parent

No specific statute found. Please read text for discussion of legal principles.

Emergency, §20–9–4.2

Minors may be treated if parental consent is not immediately available, and, in the opinion of the treating physician, the attempt to secure consent would result in delay of treatment which would threaten the minor's life or health.

*South Dakota Codified Laws (1984).

Abortion, §34–23A–7

This statute is probably unconstitutional. Please read text for discussion of constitutional principles.

Contraception

No specific statute found. Please read text for discussion of legal principles.

Sterilization

No specific statute found. Please read text for discussion of legal principles.

Sexually Transmitted Diseases, §34–23–16, §34–23–17

Any minor may consent to treatment for sexually transmitted diseases.

Substance Abuse, §34–20A–50

Any alcoholic minor may consent to treatment at an approved public treatment facility.

No specific statute found on drug abuse. Please read text for discussion of legal principles.

Mental Health, Inpatient, §27A–8–1

A person must be eighteen to consent to admission to a facility.

Mental Health, Outpatient

No specific statute found. Please read text for discussion of legal principles.

Blood Donation, §26–2–7

Seventeen-year-olds may donate blood unless the parents specifically request that such donation be prohibited.

TENNESSEE*

Age of Consent, §1–3–105(29)

The general age of majority is eighteen.

*Tennessee Code Annotated (1984).

Child with Other Adult

No specific statute found. Please read text for discussion of legal principles.

Emancipation

No specific statute found. Please read text for discussion of legal principles.

Mature Minor

No specific statute found. Please read text for discussion of legal principles.

Pregnant Minor

No specific statute found. Please read text for discussion of legal principles.

Minor Parent

No specific statute found. Please read text for discussion of legal principles.

Emergency, §63-6-222

A physician may treat a minor without parental consent where there is a good-faith belief that "delay in rendering emergency care would, to a reasonable degree of medical certainty, result in a serious threat to the life of the minor or a serious worsening of such minor's medical condition, and that emergency treatment is necessary to save the minor's life or prevent further deterioration of his condition." However, "[s]uch treatment shall be commenced only after reasonable effort is made to notify the minor's parents or guardian, if known or readily ascertainable."

Abortion, §39-4-202(f)

Minors may consent to abortions. Parental notification at least forty-eight hours prior to an abortion is required unless the minor is emancipated by marriage or the abortion must be performed sooner in order to preserve the minor's life or health.

This notification provision is most likely unconstitutional as applied to mature or emancipated minors. In addition, there are substantial questions whether the statute is constitutional as applied to immature minors, because it does not provide an alternate procedure for a determination of whether notification is in the best interests of the minor. Please read text for discussion of legal principles.

Contraception, §68–34–104, §68–34–107

It is the policy of Tennessee that contraceptive care be made available to persons without regard to age. Thus minors may consent to contraceptive care.

Sterilization, §68–34–108

A person must be eighteen or legally married to consent to sterilization. Please read the text for principles which may limit this provision.

Sexually Transmitted Diseases, §68–10–104

Minors may consent to treatment for sexually transmitted diseases.

Substance Abuse, §68–6–220

No specific statute found for alcohol abuse. Please read text for discussion of legal principles.

Any minor who abuses drugs may be treated. The provider may, but is not required to, notify the parents of treatment. This notification provision may violate federal law. See "Drug and Alcohol Records—Special Privacy Regulations" in chapter 3.

Mental Health, Inpatient, §33–6–101

Minors sixteen and over may consent to inpatient treatment.

Mental Health, Outpatient, §33–6–102

Minors sixteen and older may consent to outpatient mental health care.

Blood Donation, §68–32–101

Persons seventeen and older may donate blood on a volunteer basis only. Seventeen-year-olds may donate blood if they have had the disability of their minority removed or have obtained the written consent of their parents. But seventeen-year-olds may be accepted as blood donors in the absence of such consent if they are not compensated.

TEXAS*

Age of Consent, Family Code, T. 2, §11.01(1)

The general age of majority is eighteen.

*Texas Codes Annotated, 1985. Texas Revised Civil Statutes Annotated, 1985.

Minor with Other Adult, Family Code, T. 2, §35.01, §35.02

When the parent cannot be contacted and actual notice to the contrary has not been given by the parent, consent may be given by a grandparent; an adult brother or sister; an adult aunt or uncle; an educational institution in which the minor is enrolled; or any adult who has care and control of the minor, provided there is written authorization to do so; or any court having jurisdiction over the child. Consent by another adult must be in writing and contain the name of the minor, the name of one or both of the parents, the name of the person giving consent and his relation to the minor, a statement of the treatment to be given, and the date on which treatment is to be given.

Emancipated Minor, Family Code, T. 2, §35.03

"A minor may consent to the furnishing of hospital, medical, surgical, and dental care . . . if the minor: (1) is on active duty with the armed services . . .; (2) is 16 years of age or older and resides separate and apart from his parents . . . whether with or without the consent of the parents . . . regardless of the duration of such residence, and is managing his own financial affairs, regardless of the source of income." The provider may, but is not required to, notify parents of treatment given to or needed by the minor.

Mature Minor

No specific statute found. Please read text for discussion of legal principles.

Pregnant Minor, Family Code, T. 2, §35.03(a) (4)

Pregnant minors may consent to treatment. Notification of parents is permitted, a provision which is of suspect constitutionality. Please read text for discussion of legal principles.

Minor Parent

No specific statute found. Please read text for discussion of legal principles.

Emergency

No specific statute found. Please read text for discussion of legal principles.

Abortion, Family Code, T. 2, §35.03(a) (4)

This statute states that an unmarried minor's consent to an abortion is not sufficient.

This statute is probably unconstitutional. Please read text for discussion of constitutional principles.

Contraception

No specific statute found. Please read text for discussion of legal principles.

Sterilization

No specific statute found. Please read text for discussion of legal principles.

Sexually Transmitted Diseases, Family Code, T. 2, §35.03(a) (3)

Minors may consent to treatment for sexually transmitted diseases. The provider may, but is not required to, notify the parents.

Substance Abuse, Family Code, T. 2, §35.03(a) (6)

No specific statute found for alcohol abuse. Please read text for discussion of legal principles.

Minors may be treated for drug addiction, drug dependency, or any other condition directly related to drug use. The provider may, but is not required to, notify the parents, a provision which may conflict with federal law. (See "Drug and Alcohol Records—Special Privacy Regulations" in chapter 3.) Last, there is an apparent conflict with Health—Public, T. 71, Art. 4447i, which limits the age of treatment for drug-related conditions to minors thirteen and over.

Mental Health, Inpatient, Mental Health, T. 92, Art. 5547–22, 5547–23

Minors sixteen and over may consent to admission to a facility.

Mental Health, Outpatient

No specific statute found. Please read text for discussion of legal principles.

Blood Donation, Family Code, T. 2, §35.03 (a) (5)

A person must be eighteen to donate blood.

UTAH*

Age of Consent, §15–2–1

The general age of majority is eighteen, but all minors obtain their majority by marriage.

Child with Other Adult

No specific statute found. Please read text for discussion of legal principles.

Emancipated Adult

No specific statute found. Please read text for discussion of legal principles.

Mature Minor

No specific statute found. Please read text for discussion of legal principles.

Pregnant Minor

No specific statute found. Please read text for discussion of legal principles.

Minor Parent

No specific statute found. Please read text for discussion of legal principles.

Emergency

No specific statute found. Please read text for discussion of legal principles. Also, see §26–8–11, which relieves basic or advanced life support personnel, licensed physicians, and registered nurses from civil liability for damages resulting from omissions in delivery of emergency health care, which, presumably, would cover the failure to obtain parental consent.

Abortion, §76–7–304, §76–7–321

Minors may consent to abortions. Parental notification is required for minors who are not married, otherwise emancipated, or members of the U.S. armed forces. This notification provision is most likely unconstitu-

*Utah Code Annotated (1984).

tional as applied to mature minors or to immature minors when notification would not be in their best interests. See *H. L.* v. *Matheson*, 450 U.S. 398 (1980). Please read text for discussion of legal principles.

Contraception, §76-7-325, §76-7-321

Minors may consent to contraceptive care. Parental notification is required, whenever possible, for minors who are not married, emancipated, or members of the U.S. armed forces. This notification provision may be of questionable constitutionality as applied to mature minors. Please read text for discussion of legal principles.

Sterilization, §64-10-3

Persons must be eighteen unless married or otherwise emancipated to consent to sterilization, and the physician, through careful examination and counseling, must ensure that the person is capable of giving informed consent and, if institutionalized, has not been subjected to undue influence or coercion. Otherwise, a court order is required before a minor may be sterilized. Please read text for discussion of legal principles which may limit the rights of married or emancipated minors to consent to sterilization.

Sexually Transmitted Diseases, §26-6-18

Minors may consent to treatment for sexually transmitted diseases.

Substance Abuse

No specific statute found. Please read text for discussion of legal principles.

Mental Health, Inpatient, §64-7-29

Minors sixteen and over may consent to admission to a facility.

Mental Health, Outpatient

No specific statute found. Please read text for discussion of legal principles.

Blood Donation, §15-2-5

A person must be eighteen to consent to blood donation.

VERMONT*

Age of Consent, T. 1, §173

The general age of majority is eighteen.

Minor with Other Adult

No specific statute found. Please read text for discussion of legal principles.

Emancipated Minor

No specific statute found. Please read text for discussion of legal principles.

Mature Minor

No specific statute found. Please read text for discussion of legal principles.

Pregnant Minor

No specific statute found. Please read text for discussion of legal principles.

Minor Parent

No specific statute found. Please read text for discussion of legal principles.

Emergency

No specific statute found. Please read text for discussion of legal principles.

Abortion

No specific statute found. Please read text for discussion of legal principles.

Contraception

No specific statute found. Please read text for discussion of legal principles.

*Vermont Statutes Annotated (1984).

Sterilization

No specific statute found. Please read text for discussion of legal principles.

Sexually Transmitted Diseases, T. 18, §4226

Minors twelve and over may consent to treatment for sexually transmitted diseases. Parents must be notified if the minor requires immediate hospitalization.

Substance Abuse, T. 18, §4226

A minor over twelve may consent to treatment if found to be an alcoholic and such finding is verified by a physician.

A minor who is suspected to be dependent on drugs may consent to treatment. Parental notification is required if the minor is hospitalized. This notification provision may violate federal law. (See "Drug and Alcohol Records—Special Privacy Regulations" in chapter 3.)

Mental Health, Inpatient, T. 18, §7503

Minors fourteen and over may consent to admission to hospitals designated by the commissioner of health as adequate to provide appropriate care for the mentally ill patient.

Mental Health, Outpatient

No specific statute found. Please read text for discussion of legal principles.

Blood Donation, T. 18, §9

Seventeen-year-olds may donate blood to voluntary blood programs but may not receive compensation.

VIRGINIA*

Age of Consent, §1–13.42

The general age of majority is eighteen.

Minor with Other Adult, §54–325.2(A) (6)

A person standing *in loco parentis*, a conservator, or a guardian may consent to the medical and surgical care of a minor.

*Virginia Code (1984).

Emancipated Minor

No specific statute found. Please read text for discussion of legal principles.

Mature minor

No specific statute found. Please read text for discussion of legal principles.

Pregnant Minor, §54–325.2(D) (2)

A pregnant minor may consent to treatment.

Minor Parent

No specific statute found. Please read text for discussion of legal principles.

Emergency, §54–325.2(C)

Treatment may be provided "[w]henever delay in providing medical or surgical treatment to a minor may adversely affect such minor's recovery and no person authorized [to consent] is available within a reasonable time under the circumstances."

Consent to the treatment must be first obtained from a minor fourteen and over who is physically capable of giving consent.

Abortion, §18.2–76

Parental permission is required only when the minor has been adjudicated incompetent by a court of competent jurisdiction.

Contraception, §54–325.2(D) (2)

Minors may consent to contraceptive care.

Sterilization, §54–325.9

A person must be eighteen to consent to sterilization. Judicial authorization is required for minors between fourteen and eighteen, who cannot give informed consent.

Sexually Transmitted Diseases, §54–325.2(D) (1)

Minors may consent to treatment for sexually transmitted diseases.

Substance Abuse, §54–325.2(D) (3)

Minors may consent to medical or health services needed for the treatment or rehabilitation of substance abuse.

Mental Health, Inpatient, §37.1–65

The statute states that "any person" may consent to voluntary admission to a facility.

Mental Health, Outpatient, §54–325.2(D) (4)

Minors may consent to treatment or rehabilitation for mental illness or emotional disturbance.

Blood Donation, §54–325.2(F)

Seventeen-year-olds may donate blood to nonprofit voluntary programs but may not receive compensation.

WASHINGTON*

Age of Consent, §§26.28.010, 26.28.015

The general age of majority is eighteen.

Minor with Other Adult

No specific statute found. Please read text for discussion of legal principles.

Emancipated Minor

No specific statute found. Please read text for discussion of legal principles.

Mature Minor

No specific statute found. Please read text for discussion of legal principles.

Pregnant Minor

No specific statute found. Please read text for discussion of legal principles.

*Revised Statutes of Washington Annotated (1985).

Minor Parent, §26.28.015(5)

A minor parent may consent to care for self and child.

Emergency, §18.71.220

"No physician or hospital . . . shall be subject to civil liability, based solely upon failure to obtain consent in rendering emergency medical, surgical, hospital, or health services to any individual regardless of age where its patient is unable to give his consent for any reason and there is no other person reasonably available who is legally authorized to consent to the providing of such care: Provided, That such physician or hospital has acted in good faith and without knowledge of facts negating consent."

Abortion, §9.02.070

This statute is unconstitutional and cannot prevent mature or emancipated minors from obtaining abortions without parental consent. *State* v. *Koome*, 530 P.2d 260 (Wash. 1975). Please read text for discussion of legal principles.

Contraception

No specific statute found. Please read text for discussion of legal principles.

Sterilization

No specific statute found. Please read text for discussion of legal principles.

Sexually Transmitted Diseases, §70.24.110

Minors fourteen and over may consent to treatment for sexually transmitted diseases.

Substance Abuse, §69.54.060

Minors fourteen and older may consent to treatment for alcohol and drug abuse. The parents of a minor may not be notified, except that the minor may not become a resident of a drug treatment center without parental consent. Parents are not liable for payment unless they have joined in the consent.

Mental Health, Inpatient, §72.23.070

A person must be eighteen to consent to admission to a facility. Applications for voluntary admissions filed by parents of a minor over the age of thirteen must be accompanied by the written consent, knowingly and voluntarily given, of the minor. In addition, a voluntarily admitted minor over thirteen years of age has the right to be released on the next judicial day from the date of request unless a petition is filed in juvenile court by the professional person in charge of the facility or his designee on the grounds that the juvenile is dangerous to himself or others or that it would be in the best interests of the juvenile that he remain in the facility.

Mental Health, Outpatient

No specific statute found. Please read text for discussion of legal principles.

Blood Donation, §70.01.020

A person over eighteen may donate blood without parental consent.

WEST VIRGINIA*

Age of Consent, §2–2–10(aa)

The general age of majority is eighteen.

Minor with Other Adult

No specific statute found. Please read text for discussion of legal principles.

Emancipated Minor

No specific statute found regarding medical care, although West Virginia does have a court procedure whereby a minor may obtain a declaration of emancipation. Please read text for discussion of legal principles.

Mature Minor

No specific statute found. Please read text for discussion of legal principles.

Pregnant Minor

No specific statute found. Please read text for discussion of common law principles.

*West Virginia Code (1985).

Minor Parent

No specific statute found. Please read text for discussion of legal principles.

Emergency

No specific statute found. Please read text for discussion of legal principles.

Abortion, §16–2F–1 through 9

Parents of unemancipated minors must be given twenty-four hours' notice of the abortion, or, if the parents cannot be found after reasonable efforts, the abortion may not occur for forty-eight hours after sending them written notification. The physician must notify the minor that she may petition the circuit court for a waiver of the notification. Upon notification "being given to [the] parent . . ., the physician shall refer [the] pregnant minor to a counselor or caseworker of any church or school or of the department of human services or any other comparable agency for the purpose of arranging or accompanying [the] pregnant minor in consultation with her parents."

"Parental notification . . . may be waived by a physician, other than the physician who is to perform the abortion, if [the] other physician finds the minor mature enough to make the abortion decision independently or that notification would not be in the minor's best interest." The other physician "shall not be associated professionally or financially with the physician proposing to perform the abortion."

The pregnant minor may also petition the circuit court for a waiver if she is mature enough to make the abortion decision independently, or if parental notification would not be in her best interests.

The notification provision does not apply in emergencies where the continuation of the pregnancy constitutes an immediate threat and grave risk to the life or health of the minor and the attending physician certifies the same in writing, setting forth the threat or risk and the consequences attendant to the continuation of the pregnancy.

Contraception

No specific statute found. Please read text for discussion of legal principles.

Sterilization, §16–11–1

A person must be eighteen to consent to sterilization.

Sexually Transmitted Diseases, §16–4–10

Any minor may consent to treatment for sexually transmitted diseases.

Substance Abuse, §§60–6–23, 60A–5–504(e)

Minors may be treated for addiction to or dependence upon the use of alcoholic liquor, nonintoxicating beer, or controlled substances.

Mental Health, Inpatient, §§27–4–1, 27–4–3

Persons must be eighteen to consent to admission to a facility. Voluntary admissions are conditional upon the consent of a prospective patient who is twelve years of age or over. Patients over twelve may be released on their own regard.

Mental Health, Outpatient

No specific statute found. Please read text for discussion of legal principles.

Blood Donation, §16–21–1

A person must be eighteen to donate blood.

WISCONSIN*

Age of Consent, §48.02(2)

The general age of majority is eighteen.

Minor with Other Adult

No specific statute found. Please read text for discussion of legal principles.

Emancipated Minor

No specific statute found. Please read text for discussion of legal principles.

Mature Minor

No specific statute found. Please read text for discussion of legal principles.

Pregnant Minor

No specific statute found. Please read text for discussion of legal principles.

*Wisconsin Statutes Annotated (1984).

Minor Parent

No specific statute found. Please read text for discussion of legal principles.

Emergency

No specific statute found. Please read text for discussion of legal principles.

Abortion

No specific statute for minors found. Please read text for discussion of legal principles.

Contraception

No specific statute found. Please read text for discussion of legal principles.

Sterilization

No specific statute found. Please read text for discussion of legal principles.

Sexually Transmitted Diseases, §143.07

Any minor may consent to treatment for sexually transmitted diseases.

Substance Abuse, §51.47, §51.45

Physicians and certified health facilities may provide preventive, diagnostic, assessment, evaluation, or treatment services to minors twelve and over for abuse of alcohol or drugs. The statute requires notification of the parents of services rendered as soon thereafter as practicable. This notification provision may violate federal law. (See "Drug and Alcohol Records—Special Privacy Regulations" in chapter 3.) Also, a parent's consent is required before performing surgery unless it is essential to preserve the life or health of the minor and the parent's consent is not readily available. Parental consent is also required before administering any controlled substances to the minor, and before admitting the minor to an inpatient facility, unless admission is to detoxify the minor and will last less than seventy-two hours after the minor's admission.

Mental Health, Inpatient, §51.13

Minors fourteen or older may be voluntarily admitted if the parent so consents, or, if the parent refuses, the minor may apply to the court for permission to enter the facility.

Mental Health, Outpatient

No specific statute found. Please read text for discussion of legal principles.

Blood Donation

No specific statute found. Please read text for discussion of legal principles.

WYOMING*

Age of Consent, §14–1–101(a)

Minors may consent to health care at nineteen.

Minor with Other Adult

No specific statute found. Please read text for discussion of legal principles.

Emancipated Minor, §14–1–101(b)(iv)

"A minor may consent to health care treatment to the same extent as if he were an adult when . . . the minor is living apart from his parents . . . and is managing his own affairs regardless of his source of income."

Mature Minor

No specific statute found. Please read text for discussion of legal principles.

Pregnant Minor

No specific statute found. Please read text for discussion of legal principles.

Minor Parent

No specific statute found. Please read text for discussion of legal principles.

Emergency, §14–1–101(b)(iii)

A minor may consent to health services when the parents cannot be located with reasonable diligence "and the minor's need for health care treatment is sufficiently urgent to require immediate attention."

*Wyoming Statutes Annotated (1985).

Abortion, §35–6–101

No age is set forth for consent to an abortion. Please read text for discussion of legal principles.

Contraception

No specific statute found. Please read text for discussion of legal principles.

Sterilization

No specific statute found. Please read text for discussion of legal principles.

Sexually Transmitted Diseases, §35–4–131(a)

Any minor may consent to treatment for sexually transmitted diseases.

Substance Abuse

No specific statute found. Please read text for discussion of legal principles.

Mental Health, Inpatient, §25–10–106(a)

Persons who have reached the age of majority (nineteen) may consent to admission.

Mental Health, Outpatient

No specific statute found. Please read text for discussion of legal principles.

Blood Donation

No specific statute found. Please read text for discussion of legal principles.

Notes

Introduction

1. L. Ewald, "Medical Decision Making for Children: An Analysis of Competing Interests," 25 *St. Louis University Law Journal* 691–93 (1982).

Chapter 1: Overview

Historical Perspective: Parent–Child Relationships

1. John Locke, "Advice on Family Government" (1690), in *Children and Youth in America: A Documentary History*, vol. 1, ed. R. H. Bremner (Cambridge: Harvard University Press, 1970), pp. 132–34.
2. "Instructions for the Punishment of Incorrigible Children in Massachusetts" (1646), in *Education in the United States: A Documentary History*, vol. 1, ed. S. Cohen (New York: Random House, 1974), pp. 370–71.
3. J. F. Kett, *Rites of Passage: Adolescence in America, 1970 to the Present* (New York: Basic Books, 1977), chapter 1.
4. See, for example, New York General Obligations Law, §3–109.

5. "The Mental Hygiene Movement," in Bremner, *Children and Youth in America*, vol. 2 (1971), pp. 1040–57.
6. Ibid., "Issues and Trends in Education," pp. 1420–29.
7. Santosky v. Kramer, 455 U.S. 745 (1982).
8. In re Gault, 387 U.S. 1 (1967).
9. Schall v. Martin, 104 S.Ct. 2403 (1984).
10. Tinker v. Des Moines Independent School District, 393 U.S. 503 (1969).
11. See, for example, Ingraham v. Wright, 430 U.S. 651 (1977): corporal punishment within school setting held constitutional; Parham v. J.R., 442 U.S. 584 (1979): parents allowed to commit child to mental facility over child's objection as long as certain minimal due process procedures observed.
12. Roe v. Wade, 410 U.S. 113 (1973); Doe v. Bolton, 410 U.S. 179 (1973).
13. Planned Parenthood v. Danforth, 428 U.S. 52 (1976).
14. Bellotti v. Baird, 443 U.S. 622 (1979).

Definition of Law

1. Roe v. Wade, 410 U.S. 113 (1973).
2. Plessy v. Ferguson, 163 U.S. 537 (1896).
3. Brown v. Board of Education, 347 U.S. 483 (1954).
4. See 42 U.S.C. §300(a) as amended.
5. Planned Parenthood v. Heckler, 712 F.2d 650 (D.C. Cir. 1983).
6. American Psychiatric Association, *The Principles of Medical Ethics* (Washington, D.C., 1981), rev. ed., p. 3.
7. See, for example, Griswold v. Connecticut, 381 U.S. 479 (1965).

Informed Consent

1. A. Rosoff, *Informed Consent: A Guide for Health Care Providers* (Rockville, Md.: Aspen Publication, 1981); J. Katz, *The Silent World of Doctor and Patient* (New York: The Free Press, 1984).
2. Schloendorff v. New York Hospital, 211 N.Y. 125, 129–30 (1914).
3. Katz, *Silent World*, p. 60.
4. Rosoff, *Informed Consent*, p. 41.
5. See, for example, New York Public Health Law, §2805–d(4).
6. Darrah v. Kite, 301 N.Y.S.2d 286 (App. Div., 3rd Dept., 1969).
7. 139 N.E.2d 25 (Ohio 1956).
8. 469 P.2d 330 (Kansas 1970).
9. 108 N.W. 94, 96 (Mich. 1906).
10. Rosoff, *Informed Consent*, pp. 188–89.

Right to Privacy and Parental Notification

1. Roe v. Wade, 410 U.S. 113 (1973).
2. Griswold v. Connecticut, 381 U.S. 479 (1965); Eisenstadt v. Baird, 405 U.S. 438 (1972); Skinner v. Oklahoma, 316 U.S. 535 (1942).
3. Loving v. Virginia, 388 U.S. 1 (1967).
4. Whalen v. Roe, 429 U.S. 589 (1977).
5. Ibid.
6. See, for example, Arkansas Statutes, §82–632.
7. See, for example, New York Penal Law, §265.25.
8. See, for example, Idaho Code, §16–1619.
9. Tarasoff v. Regents of the University of California, 551 P.2d 334 (Cal. 1976).
10. See, for example, Oregon Revised Statutes, §109.650.
11. See, for example, Florida Statutes Annotated, §743.064(3).
12. See, for example, Annotated Laws of Massachusetts, C.112, §12F.

Chapter 2: Law According to Patient Status

Minors Accompanied by a Parent

1. Record of the Association of the Bar of the City of New York, "The Medical Treatment of Minors Under New York Law" (December 1976), p. 700.

Minors Accompanied by Adults Other Than Parents

1. Moss v. Rishworth, 222 S.W. 225 (Tex. Comm'n App. 1920).
2. Bakker v. Welsh, 108 N.W. 94 (Mich. 1906).
3. Bonner v. Moran, 126 F.2d 121 (D.D.C. 1941).
4. See, for example, Arkansas and Georgia.
5. Moss at 226.
6. Bonner at 122–23.
7. Bakker at 635–36.

Minors in Boarding Schools, Camps, and Related Institutions

1. Record of the Association of the Bar of the City of New York, "The Medical Treatment of Minors Under New York Law" (December 1976), p. 704.

Age of Consent

1. Amendment 26 was adopted on July 5, 1971.

2. New York General Obligations Law, §3–101.
3. New York Penal Law, §130.05(3).
4. New York Alcohol Beverage Control Law, §65–b.
5. New York Penal Law, §10(18).
6. New York Domestic Relations Law, §32.
7. See, for example, Louisiana Statutes Annotated, 40: §1299.53.

Emancipated Minors

1. 431 P.2d 719 (Wash. 1967).
2. Everett v. Sherfey, 1 Iowa 356 (1855).
3. Hunycutt & Co. v. Thompson, 74 S.E. 628 (N.C. 1912).
4. Poudre Valley Hospital District v. Heckart, 491 P.2d 984 (1971); Timmerman v. Brown, 233 S.E.2d 106 (S.C. 1977); Carter v. Cangello, 164 Cal. Rptr. 361 (1980).
5. Accent Service Co. v. Ebsen, 306 N.W.2d 575 (Neb. 1981).
6. See, for example, Alaska Statutes, §09.65.100(1); Massachusetts General Laws, 112 §12F; Texas Family Code, §35.03.
7. Ross v. Department of Public Welfare, 431 A.2d 1135 (Pa. 1981).
8. A. Holder, *Legal Issues in Pediatrics and Adolescent Medicine* (New York: John Wiley & Sons, 1977), p. 139.
9. See, for example, Alabama, Arizona, California, District of Columbia, Florida, Georgia, Hawaii, Idaho, Illinois, Indiana, and Iowa in state-by-state table.
10. See, for example, Alaska in state-by-state table.

Other Minors Away from Home

1. National Inspection Program, Department of Health and Human Services, Office of Inspector General, *Runaway and Homeless Youth* (October 1983), p. 4.
2. A. Holder, *Legal Issues in Pediatrics and Adolescent Medicine* (New York: John Wiley & Sons, 1977), p. 140.
3. Ibid.
4. Ibid., pp. 139–40.

Minor Parents

1. See, for example, Meyer v. Nebraska, 262 U.S. 390 (1923); Pierce v. Society of Sisters, 268 U.S. 510 (1925); Wisconsin v. Yoder, 406 U.S. 205 (1972); Santosky v. Kramer, 455 U.S. 745 (1982).
2. Mississippi, §41–41–3.
3. Caban v. Mohammed, 441 U.S. 380 (1979).

Mature Minors

1. Bach v. Long Island Jewish Hospital, 267 N.Y.S.2d 289 (Sup. Ct. Nassau Co. 1966).
2. Younts v. St. Francis Hospital and School of Nursing, 469 P.2d 330 (Kan. 1970).
3. Lacey v. Laird, 139 N.E.2d 25 (Ohio 1956).
4. Bonner v. Moran, 126 F.2d 121 (D.D.C. 1941).
5. Bach at 291.
6. Younts at 338.
7. A. Holder, *Legal Issues in Pediatrics and Adolescent Medicine* (New York: John Wiley & Sons, 1977), p. 130. See also H. Pilpel, "Minors' Rights to Medical Care," 36 *Albany Law Review* 466 (1972).
8. Lacey at 34 (Judge Taft concurring).
9. Bonner at 123.
10. W. Wadlington, "Minors and Health Care: The Age of Consent," 11 *Osgoode Hall Law Journal* 119–20 (1973).

Chapter 3: Law According to Patient Need

Emergency, Urgent, and/or Necessary Health Care

1. Wells v. McGehee, 39 So.2d 196 (La. Ct. App. 1949).
2. Sullivan, et al. v. Montgomery, 279 N.Y.S. 575 (City Ct. 1935).
3. Jackovach v. Yocum, 237 N.W. 444 (Iowa 1931).
4. Luka v. Lowrie, et al., 136 N.W. 1106 (Mich. 1912).
5. Arizona Revised Statutes Annotated, §36–2271(C).
6. Virginia Code, §54–325.2(C).
7. North Dakota Statutes, §14–10–17.1.
8. Zoski v. Gaines, 260 N.W. 99 (Mich. 1935).
9. Moss v. Rishworth, 222 S.W. 225 (Tex. Comm'n App. 1920).
10. Dewes v. Indian Health Services, 504 F. Supp. 203 (D.S.D. 1980).
11. Tabor v. Scobee, 254 S.W.2d 474 (Ken. 1953).
12. Arizona Revised Statutes Annotated, §36–2271(C).
13. Tennessee Code Annotated, §63–6–222.
14. Florida Statutes Annotated, §743.064(3).
15. Ibid.

Contraception

1. Carey v. Population Services International, 431 U.S. 678 (1977).

2. 42 U.S.C. §§ 602(a)(15) and 1396a(a)(4)(C) and 8; 42 C.F.R. §220.21; 42 U.S.C. §3000 *et seq.*
3. T—H— v. Jones, 425 F. Supp. 873 (D. Utah 1975) (3 judge court), *aff'd sub nom*, Jones v. T—H—, 425 U.S. 986 (1976); National Family Planning and Reproductive Health v. Heckler, 559 F. Supp. 658 (D.D.C. 1983).

Abortion

1. Roe v. Wade, 410 U.S. 113 (1973).
2. Harris v. McRae, 448 U.S. 297 (1980).
3. Moe v. Secretary of Administration and Finance, 417 N.E.2d 387 (Mass. 1981); Committee to Defend Reproductive Rights v. Myers, 625 P.2d 779 (Cal. 1981).
4. See City of Akron v. Akron Center for Reproductive Health, 103 S. Ct. 2481 (1983); Planned Parenthood v. Ashcroft, 103 S. Ct. 2517 (1983); Simopoulos v. Virginia, 103 S. Ct. 2532 (1983).
5. Roe at 154.
6. Roe at 164.
7. Roe at 163.
8. Ibid.
9. Ibid.
10. City of Akron at 2507 (dissenting opinion of Justice O'Connor).
11. Planned Parenthood of Missouri v. Danforth, 428 U.S. 52, 73 (1976).
12. Danforth at 75.
13. Danforth at 74.
14. Bellotti v. Baird, 443 U.S. 622, 643–44 (1979).
15. Bellotti at 644.
16. H. L. v. Matheson, 450 U.S. 398 (1981).
17. In re Smith, 295 A.2d 238 (Md. 1972); Ballard v. Anderson, 484 P.2d 1345 (Cal. 1971); Comment, "Minor's Right to Refuse Court-Ordered Abortions," 7 *Suffolk University Law Review* 1157 (1973).
18. Matter of Barbara C., 474 N.Y.S. 2d 799 (2nd Dept. 1984).

Sterilization

1. 42 C.F.R. §50.203 (1984); 42 C.F.R. §§441.253, 254 (1984).
2. Smith v. Seibly, 431 P.2d 719 (Wash. 1967).
3. In re Grady, 426 A.2d 467, 472 (N.J. 1981).
4. Skinner v. Oklahoma, 316 U.S. 535, 541 (1942).
5. See, for example, Guardianship of Tully, 83 Cal. App. 3d 698 (Cal. Ct. App. 1978); Matter of S.C.E., 378 A.2d 144 (Del. 1977); A. L. v. G. R.

H., 325 N.E.2d 501 (Ind. Ct. App. 1975), cert. denied, 425 U.S. 936 (1976); In re D. D., 394 N.Y.S.2d 139 (Surr. Ct. Nassau Co. 1977), aff'd on other grounds, 408 N.Y.S.2d 104 (App. Div. 2nd Dept. 1978).

6. Stump v. Sparkman, 435 U.S. 349 (1978); Wentzel V. Montgomery General Hospital, 447 A.2d 1244 (Md. 1982); In re Grady, 426 A.2d 467 (N.J. 1981); Matter of C. D. M., 627 P.2d 607 (Alaska 1981); Matter of Guardianship of Hayes, 608 P.2d 635 (Wash. 1980) (en banc); In re Penny N., 414 A.2d 541 (N.H. 1980); Matter of A. W. 637 P.2d 366 (Colo. 1981) (en banc); Matter of Sallmaier, 378 N.Y.S.2d 989 (Sup. Ct. Queen Co. 1976).

7. Hayes at 637.

8. Factors derived from cases set forth in footnote 7.

Substance Abuse

1. Stern, "Medical Treatment and the Teenager," 7 *Clearinghouse Review* 1 (1973).

2. See, for example, Delaware, Kansas, Ohio, South Dakota, and Tennessee in state-by-state table.

3. See, for example, California, Illinois, and Mississippi in state-by-state table.

4. A. Holder, *Legal Issues in Pediatrics and Adolescent Medicine* (New York: John Wiley & Sons, 1977), pp. 142–143.

5. See, for example, Connecticut and Iowa in state-by-state table.

6. See, for example, California, Maine, and Kentucky in state-by-state table.

7. See, for example, Illinois in state-by-state table.

8. See, for example, Montana in state-by-state table.

Drug and Alcohol Records—Special Privacy Regulations

1. 42 C.F.R., §2 et seq (1984).

2. 42 C.F.R. §2.11(i) (1984).

3. 42 C.F.R. §2.11(o) (1984).

4. 42 C.R.F. §2.13 (1984).

5. 55 N.Y.2d 588 (1982).

6. Ibid., p. 590.

7. 42 C.F.R., §2.15 (1984).

8. 42 C.F.R. §§2.33, 2.35–37 (1984).

9. 42 C.F.R. §2.31 (1984).

10. 42 C.F.R. §2.40 (1984).

11. 42 C.F.R. §§2.51–52 (1984).

12. Legal Action Center of the City of New York, "Confidentiality and Child Abuse: An Update," *Of Substance*, September/October, 1984.
13. Ibid.
14. 42 C.F.R. §§2.62–63 (1984).
15. 42 C.F.R. §2.64 (1984).
16. 42 C.F.R. §2.65 (1984).
17. 42 C.F.R. §2.66 (1984).

Mental Health Care

1. Parham v. J. R., 442 U.S. 584 (1979).
2. Ibid.
3. Caesar v. Mountanos, 542 F.2d 1064, 1071–72 (9th Cir. 1976) (Hufstedler, J., dissenting).
4. Hawaii Psychiatric Society, District Branch of the American Psychiatric Association v. Ariyoshi, 481 F. Supp. 1028 (D. Hawaii 1979).
5. Youngberg v. Romeo, 475 U.S. 307 (1982); Rennie v. Klein, 653 F.2d 836 (3rd Cir. 1981), remanded, 458 U.S. 1119 (1982); Rogers v. Okin, 634 F.2d 650 (1st Cir. 1980), vacated and remanded, Mills v. Rogers, 457 U.S. 291 (1982).

Chapter 4: Special Situations

Minors as Research Subjects

1. Research regulations for adults, as revised, were issued on January 26, 1981. The regulations for children were finally published by HHS on March 8, 1983, and became effective on June 6, 1983. See 45 C.F.R. 46, Subpart D.
2. 45 C.F.R. §46.101(a) (1984).
3. 45 C.F.R. §46.102(e) (1984).
4. The National Commission for the Protection of Human Subjects of Biomedical and Behavioral Research, *The Belmont Report: Ethical Principles and Guidelines for the Protection of Human Subjects of Research*, DHEW Publication, No. (03) 77–004 (Washington, D.C., 1977), p. 3.
5. Ibid.
6. Ibid.
7. 45 C.F.R. §46.101(b) (1984).
8. 45 C.F.R. §§46.108–113 (1984).
9. 45 C.F.R. §46.116 (1984).

10. 45 C.F.R. §46.408 (a), (b) (1984).
11. 45 C.F.R. §46.408(c) (1984).
12. Ibid.
13. The National Commission for the Protection of Human Subjects of Biomedical and Behavioral Research, *Research Involving Children: Report and Recommendations*, DHEW Publication No. COS 777–004, (Washington, D.C., 1977), quoted in R. Levine, "Research Involving Children: An Interpretation of the New Regulations," *IRB*, vol. 5, no. 4, July/August 1983, p. 2.
14. 45 C.F.R. §46.402 (a) (1984).
15. For a discussion of questionnaires generally, see A. R. Holder, "Case Study: Teenagers and Questionnaire Research," *IRB*, vol. 5, no. 3, May/June 1983.
16. Levine, "Research Involving Children," p. 2. See also A. R. Holder, "Can Teenagers Participate in Research Without Parental Consent?" and R. M. Veatch, "Commentary: Beyond Consent to Treatment," both in *IRB*, vol. 3, no. 2, February 1981.
17. 45 C.F.R. §46.402(a) (1984).
18. Levine, "Research Involving Children," p. 1.
19. 45 C.F.R. §46.408(a) (1984).
20. 45 C.F.R. §46.402(b) (1984).
21. 45 C.F.R. §46.408(a) (1984).
22. 45 C.F.R. §46.406(a) (1984).
23. 45 C.F.R. §46.406(b) (1984).
24. Levine, "Research Involving Children," p. 3.
25. 45 C.F.R. §46.406(c) (1984).
26. 45 C.F.R. §46.405 (1984).
27. 45 C.F.R. §46.116(e) (1984).

Parental Refusal of Treatment for a Minor Child

1. In re Sampson, 29 N.Y.2d 900 (1972).
2. Matter of Hofbauer, 47 N.Y.2d 648 (1979).
3. Weber v. Stony Brook Hospital, 60 N.Y.2d 208 (1983).
4. Weber at 212.
5. Randolph v. City of New York, *N.Y.L.J.*, Oct. 12, 1984, p. 6, col. 4 (N.Y. App. Term).
6. D. Bross, *Child Abuse and Neglect*, Vol. 6 (Pergamon Press, 1982), pp. 375–81.
7. Matter of Hamilton, 657 S.W.2d 425 (Tenn. 1983).

Care of Handicapped Newborns

1. 29 U.S.C., §794; 45 C.F.R. §84.61 (1984).
2. American Academy of Pediatrics v. Heckler, 561 F. Supp. 395 (D.D.C. 1983); United States v. University Hospital, 575 F. Supp. 607 (E.D.N.Y. 1983), aff'd 729 F.2d 144 (2d Cir. 1984).
3. 49 Fed. Reg. 48,160 (1984) (proposed Dec. 10, 1984).
4. Ibid., p. 48,161.
5. Ibid., p. 48,163.

Parent–Child Conflict

1. In re Hudson, 126 P.2d 765 (Wash. 1942).
2. Hudson at 768.
3. Hudson at 778.
4. L. Ewald, "Medical Decision Making for Children: An Analysis of Competing Interests," 25 *St. Louis University Law Journal* 705 (1982),; In re Green, 292 A.2d 387 (Pa. 1972), remanded to trail court, 292 A.2d 279 (Pa. 1973), aff'g on remand.
5. In re Seiferth, 309 N.Y. 80, 84 (1955).
6. Seiferth at 84.
7. Seiferth at 85.

Organ Donation

1. Donation permitted in Strunk v. Strunk, 445 S.W.2d 145 (Ky. 1969); Little v. Little, 576 S.W.2d 493 (Tex. Civ. App. 1978); Hart v. Brown, 289 A.2d 386 (Conn. Super. Ct. 1972). For a discussion of the Massachusetts cases, see A. Holder, *Legal Issues in Pediatrics and Adolescent Medicine* (New York: John Wiley & Sons, 1977), p. 175.
2. Donation not permitted in In re Richardson, 284 So.2d 185 (La. Ct. App. 1973); In re Guardianship of Pescinski, 226 N.W.2d 180 (Wis. 1975).
3. See cases cited in note 1.
4. See cases cited in note 2.
5. Holder, *Legal Issues*, pp. 175–78.

Chapter 5: Confidentiality and Health Care Records

The Health Record Privacy Dilemma

1. *Psychiatric Opinion*, vol. 12, no. 1, Jan. 1975: Special Issue in Health Record Privacy.

2. A. Hofmann, "Is Confidentiality in Health Care Records a Pediatric Concern?," *Pediatrics*, 57 (Feb. 1976)2:pp. 170–72.

New Directions in Health Record Privacy Legislation

1. 5 U.S.C. §552a.
2. 45 C.F.R. Part 5b (1984).
3. 20 U.S.C. §1232g; 34 C.F.R. §§99.1 et seq. (1984).

Information Release Without Patient or Parental Consent

1. *Personal Privacy in an Information Society: The Report of the Privacy Protection Study Commission*, July 1977, pp. 277–317, U.S. Government Printing Office, Washington, D.C. (stock #052-003-00395-3).

Management of the Health Record

1. A. Westin., *Medical Records: Should Patients Have Access?*, The Hastings Center Report, New York, Dec. 1977, pp. 23–28.
2. A. Westin, *Medical Records: Should Patients Have Access?*, at p. 27.
3. E. Stern, R. Furedy, and M. J. Simonton, "Patient Access to Medical Records on a Psychiatric Inpatient Unit," *American Journal of Psychiatry*, 136 (3): March, 1979, pp. 327–29.

Chapter 6: Strategic Issues and Problem Situations

The Payment Question

1. 42 Am. Jur.2d *Infants* §65 (1985).
2. Myers v. Hodge, 42 S.E.2d 23 (1947).
3. See Southern Railway Co. v. Neeley, 114 S.E.2d 283 (Ga. Ct. App. 1960); Hagerman v. Mutual Hospital Insurance, Inc., 371 N.E.2d 394 (Ind. Ct. App. 1978).
4. An exception may be carved out for emergency health care and the law may presume that the parent consented to the health care. For another exception, see Revised Statutes of Nebraska, §71–1121 (parents liable for VD treatment given to minor child).

Index

NOTE: Entries for statutes of individual states refer to material found in chapters 1 through 6 only. For specific legal information regarding any state or the District of Columbia, the reader should also check the Appendix table.